DOCTORS IN COMMUNITY

DOCTORS IN COMMUNITY

The Training of Interns and Residents
at Brackenridge Hospital, Austin, Texas

CHRISTOPHER S. CHENAULT, MD

Copyright © 2017 by Christopher S. Chenault, MD.

Library of Congress Control Number: 2017908556
ISBN: Hardcover 978-1-5434-2715-8
Softcover 978-1-5434-2714-1
eBook 978-1-5434-2713-4

All rights reserved. No part of this book may be reproduced or transmitted in any form or by any means, electronic or mechanical, including photocopying, recording, or by any information storage and retrieval system, without permission in writing from the copyright owner.

Any people depicted in stock imagery provided by Thinkstock are models, and such images are being used for illustrative purposes only.
Certain stock imagery © Thinkstock.

Print information available on the last page.

Rev. date: 08/04/2017

To order additional copies of this book, contact:
Xlibris
1-888-795-4274
www.Xlibris.com
Orders@Xlibris.com
762367

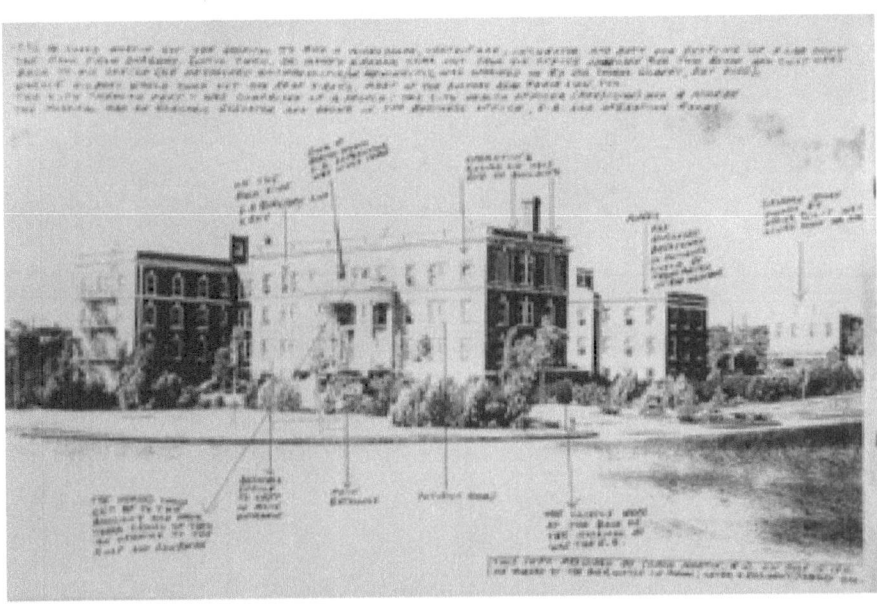

CONTENTS

Dedication ix
Introduction..1
History of Medical Training in the US and Texas 5
Brackenridge Begins a Training Program: The first Interns 9
Medicine in the 1930's 16
The War Years..24
The Growth Years of the 1950's and 60's...31
Progress in Organization 48
The 1970's, The Perfect Storm 57
Central Texas Medical Foundation..66
Ambulance Service...69
Improving the Emergency Room..74
A New Training Program 87
Pediatrics..88
Internal Medicine...100
Surgery Department.. 111
Obstetrics and Gynecology..122
Family Medicine 134
Psychiatry Department... 147
Pathology 151
Transitional years of the early 21st Century..................................... 155
Creating a Medical School 165
Footnotes 169
Appendix A... 173
Appendix B..225
Appendix C: Articles of Incorporation for CTMF.......................227

Dedication

This book is dedicated to the many doctors in the Travis County Medical Society who have served the many patients who have come to Brackenridge Hospital and who have made the training of interns and residents possible over the past 85 years. They have worked endless hours to serve their community and to make it a better place in which to live.

Introduction

Austin, Texas has a great tradition of medical excellence. In this writing it is my goal to demonstrate the qualities that led a community of doctors to nurture young doctors, fresh out of medical school, to become better practitioners and better people, as they care for their patients. The choices that they made to spend time beyond their own practices to make sure that these trainees "learned the ropes" speaks volumes about their character and drive. These characteristics, seen in many over generations, reflect a special kind of person who gives of himself or herself with no idea that anyone will recognize their efforts or reward them for the hours that they have spent. For the first forty years of this history there was minimal organization or supervising structure, and just a will to improve quality. For the next forty years there developed a significant progression of well thought out organizations that were able to respond to the complex requirements of the national medical organizations as well as community, state, and federal regulations to make the system even more responsive. There has been a progression of teaching techniques from the older "follow the masters" approach to the modern "evidence based medicine" process of today.

Entwined in the many details of creating a more organized training program was the significant effort to provide more medical services to the community. This involved the creation of a new hospital building, a new emergency room with a different form of management, and a completely new emergency medical/ambulance service. This effort was bolstered by the election of Dr. Bud Dryden to the City Council in 1971 and his attempt to put more pressure on the process of completing the new hospital building and creating the emergency medical service.

The history of the training program for interns and residents at Brackenridge Hospital in Austin, Texas, reflects a continuum of ideas that have changed with time and with different regulations created by national accreditation organizations. In that story, there are many choices that have been made by a large number of dedicated doctors who have contributed much to the community. There were many who chose to spend time, and sometimes a lot of time, doing something that would contribute to improvements in the community of medicine rather than their own individual interests. In the early years, local doctors chose to take interns under their wing to nurture them along because they liked to do it. There were some pioneers, like Dr. Raleigh Ross and Dr. Bud Dryden, who saw that things could be better and chose to organize the training program and get it accredited so that they could attract better candidates. They hoped that some of those better doctors would stay in Austin. The hours they spent are somewhat off the charts of dedication. Dr. Georgia Legett chose to reach out to the University of Texas Medical Branch at Galveston to initiate an obstetrics program in Austin with residents from Galveston. She followed through as the program started and would teach in the clinics and assist the residents with their more difficult cases. She also recruited other doctors to help in this process. Dr. Maurice Hood chose to start a cardiac and vascular surgery program that would lead to development of an intensive care unit, respiratory care equipment, and trained technicians, and push other hospitals to a new level of cardiac surgery and patient intensive care units. Drs. Jack Moncreif and Jonathan Dechard decided to spend time training students and residents from Galveston in nephrology, and then chose to spend a lot more time working with the new Central Texas Medical Foundation (CTMF) to organize an internal medicine residency program. The choice to spend hours working with the board of the Travis County Medical Society, the new board of the CTMF, and the various department chairmen in creating the new organized training program is remarkable. These were hours they could have spent at the lake or at home or reading a book but they chose to contribute to the community. Just as Dr. Hood's choices led to new intensive care units across this community, early trainee Dr. Claud Martin's request for more laboratory equipment led to better patient evaluations, and Dr. Moncreif"s drive led to kidney transplants. The choices made by many through the years to enhance the learning experience for interns and residents in Austin created the fertile ground that would nurture a new medical school in Austin in 2015.

I found it interesting that some trainees chose Austin in the early years, even though the community was untested as a center for a training program. There were some doctors who returned to Austin because it was their home. There were many more who chose to come because it is an attractive place to live. And there were a number who came to this training program because they were assured of seeing lots of patient pathology and would be able to work with community doctors.

History of Medical Training in the US and Texas

The American Medial Association was founded in 1847. That same year they formed the Committee on Medical Education that created standards for a medical education at the time. In 1904 they took another step in a campaign to raise the educational requirements for physicians. In 1910, the American Medical Association and the Carnegie Foundation sponsored a report that reviewed medical education at schools across the country. That report, referred to as the Flexner Report, documented some dismal centers of medical education in a number of places including Wisconsin and Chicago, They also published the "Essentials of an Acceptable Medical College." That has been revised with upgrades eight times in the ensuing years. A number of schools, including several considered diploma mills, closed after the Flexner report was published. In 1914 the standards for an internship were published and in 1923 the standards for medical specialty training, or residency, were established.[1]

In 1891, the first medical school in Texas, The University of Texas Medical Branch (UTMB), was opened in Galveston with one building and a class of fewer than 50 students. This was accomplished after 10 years of political infighting for a location and concerns about finances. The Flexner report of 1910 concluded that UTMB was the only school in Texas "fit to continue the work of training physicians."

The John Sealy Hospital in Galveston opened in 1890 as the new city hospital supported by $50,000 from the estate of John Sealy, who had left the money for a public charity. The hospital was administered by the city of Galveston through a board until 1941 when it came under the complete control of the University of Texas Medial Branch.

In 1884, six years before the hospital in Galveston, the City of Austin and the Travis County Commissioners, jointly built a hospital on the city block originally designated for a hospital in the survey of the City by Edwin Waller in 1839. This block was placed in the northeast part of the city, a block at the intersection of 15th Street and East Avenue, so that the prevailing wind from the south would blow any bad airs or humors of illness away from town and to the north and east. Forty-five years after the survey, the hospital became a reality in an atmosphere of public concern about the need for such a facility and the general bad reputation of hospitals as pest houses. Sterile technique was little understood at that time. Most individuals were cared for in their homes and thus, in retrospect, limited the contamination of one patient from another. Hospitals, where many poor came for care, required patients to be in closer proximity to each other. The spread of disease and the contamination of wounds was higher in many hospitals than at home. Thus, there was a significant fear of being admitted to hospitals because one might catch another illness.

Nevertheless the need for a facility in Austin, where the acutely ill could be cared for, was a growing concern. This was especially true with the recent closing of a private hospital called the Austin City Infirmary. It was closed for financial reasons. At the time, the City provided for indigent care by hiring a city physician who would care for private patients but would also care for the poor under a contract. With the addition of the city hospital there was a central place for patient care. The City physician came to the hospital weekly on rounds and discussed patients with the resident physician who lived at the hospital and provided daily care, along with the matron or "housemother" who kept up with the supplies.

With time and improved medical care, along with improved financial management and not a little promotion by the local newspaper, the hospital, called City/County hospital, became more accepted by the community and the local doctors. The city limited the admission of patients with infectious disease in an effort to rid the facility of the name "pest house." In the late nineteenth century, medicine in general was improving in the fields of surgery, anesthesia techniques, and the use of more standardized medications. In 1902, The "Biologics Control

Act," was passed by the congress to ensure the purity and safety of serums, vaccines, and similar products used to prevent or treat diseases.[2] The government limited patent medications and pharmacists could no longer prescribe drugs. The act of writing prescriptions was left to physicians who had more clinical experience. A series of Congressional acts and legal actions before the courts regulated drugs and patented medications in the early 1900's.

In 1907 the county commissioners decided they no longer wanted to support the hospital. The city fathers could not convince them otherwise, so, much to the consternation of those city leaders, the hospital became the responsibility of the City of Austin. With continued growth of Austin, more hospital beds were needed. Under the influence of Dr. Robert John Brackenridge, (1839-1918) a doctor and wealthy businessman, and after much wrangling over several years, a new red brick hospital was built facing East Avenue. Interestingly, a few months after the rejection of a petition to build a separate new county hospital, the new City Hospital building was opened. Dr. Brackenridge became the chairman of the board.

In 1929, the new south wing was added, providing a total of 70 beds, and remodeling provided new operating rooms. About that time a name change was discussed. The primary reason for the change was to give a new image to the City Hospital. After some months of debate, the hospital was renamed Brackenridge Hospital, partially because many of the doctors and the general citizens referred to it by that name already, but also because of the extensive involvement of Dr. Brackenridge in its history and promotion. The oldest public hospital in Texas, Brackenridge is also unique in that most public hospitals are county hospitals and not owned or managed by a city.[3]

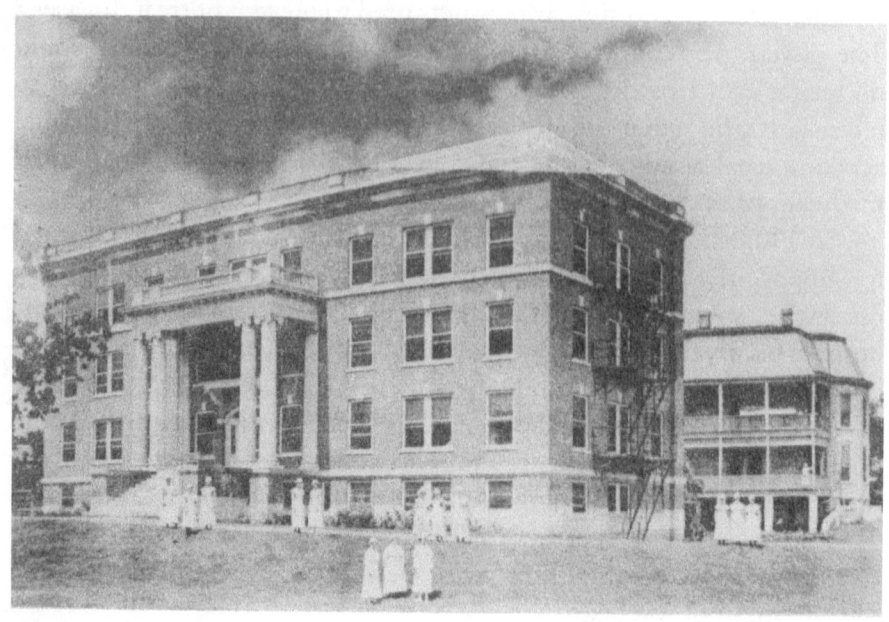

Front view of City County Hospital, brick (with permission: Austin History Center, Austin Public Library.)

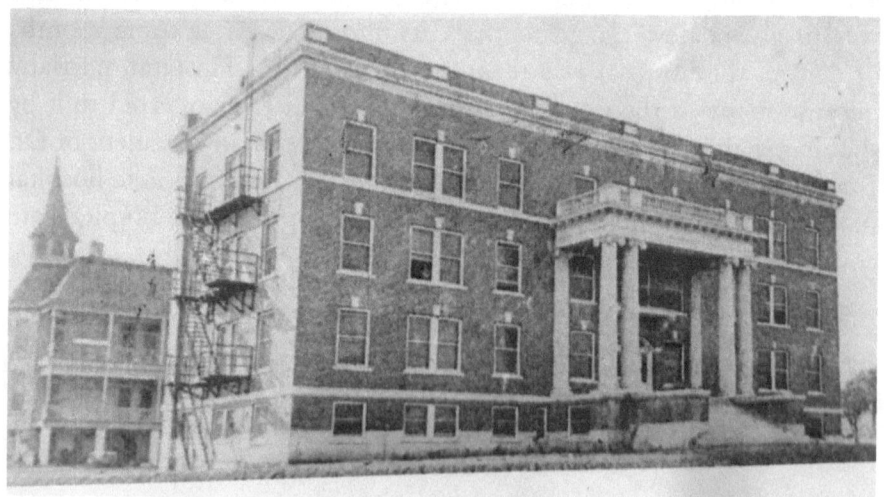

Old red brick building facing East Avenue with wood original hospital structure behind. (with permission, Austin History Center, Austin Public Library.)

Brackenridge Begins a Training Program: The first Interns

Dr. George Edmund Bennack

In 1931, the first intern presented for training at Brackenridge hospital from June 4, 1931, to July 15, 1932. Dr. George Edmund Bennack, M. D. graduated from the University of Texas Medical Branch at Galveston. It is interesting to ponder how he came to choose Austin as a place for further training. As internships had been formally defined by the American Medical Association only 17 years earlier and most doctors started practice right out of medical school, his choice to study an extra year was uncommon but becoming more prevalent. At that time, internships in Galveston did not pay anything except meals, laundry and what the few insurance companies paid for hospital care, divided among the house staff. Most internships paid about ten dollars per month but Brackenridge, trying to attract a new program, must have felt $50 per month would be more competitive. It is assumed that the administrator of the hospital, Mr. M. W. Bralley, was involved in this process and put a notice at the medical school in Galveston. The pay would have been significant because Dr. Bennack was older than most of his classmates, married and had one child while in medical school. His wife and child did not come with him to Austin. According to Mary Micka of the Medical Services and Education office at Brackenridge, who interviewed Dr. Bennack in 1991, the pay was the element on which he made his decision. In addition to the salary, he received room and board and laundry services. He was the only intern at the time and was on call 24 hours per day 7 days a week. As he lived at the hospital, he was called frequently to the emergency room. He also saw the hospitalized patients. There were no specialty floors and the only division of patients was between Negroes in the annex and white patients in the main hospital.[4]

Dr. Bennack's primary supervisor was Dr. Lee Edens, the city health officer or city physician. As city physician, Dr. Edens had a number of responsibilities. He saw or supervised the care of poor people. As Brackenridge had grown over the years, the care of the poor became more centralized at the hospital that now had 70 beds. Dr. Edens had a private practice but also saw the poor in his office. Dr. Bennack would call on Dr. Edens "any time he was needed" to see patients in the ER or on the hospital floors. Dr. Edens had been the resident physician at Brackenridge for a year in 1928. He then took on the job of city physician from 1929 to 1934.

Dr. E. O. Chemine became the resident doctor at Brackenridge following Dr. Edens and remained in that position until 1934. He would have been a resource for Dr. Bennack. 4. The community doctors provided a great deal of the teaching for Dr. Bennack, as well as direct patient care. According to Mary Micka's interview, Dr. Ben Epright was a dermatologist and staffed the skin clinic. Dr. Claud Meiars was an ear, nose and throat doctor and helped in the ENT clinic. He also did the tonsillectomies. Dr. Henry Hilgartner, Jr. was the ophthalmologist and ran the eye clinic. Dr. Bennack recalled, "being reprimanded when he had a patient with a severe eye injury, got the socket all cleaned out, and thought he had done a good job." Dr. Hilgartner "may have thought so too, but put him in his place for not calling for help." The following story suggests that Dr. Bennack scrubbed with all of these doctors as time permitted. He was supposed to scrub with the surgeon, Dr. Howard Grandberry on an appendectomy. Instead of scrubbing with Dr. Bennack, Dr. Grandberry "told him to go ahead, as he knew he could do it" by himself. Dr. Benneck also did surgery quite often with his "chief" Dr. Edens.[5]

In addition to help from these doctors, he was supported by Dr. Caroline Crowell, a general practitioner who also ran the University of Texas Student Health Center. She lived at Brackenridge hospital and "had a room on the second floor over the emergency room." "When an emergency came in, she would hear it and go down to help out."

When there was some down time on the schedule, Dr. Bennack and Dr. Crowell would go across the street to the tennis courts to play. Since it was close, the staff could run over and call them when needed back at the hospital. Again, according to Mary Micka's interview, Dr. Bennack felt his year as an intern "was very pleasant." "The only information found regarding his internship in the hospital's records is from a personnel card that verified his dates of training and remarked "services have been excellent.""

The records at the hospital contain a letter, dated 1953, to the Chairman of the Credentials Committee at Valley Baptist Hospital in Harlingen. Harlingen is about 20 miles south of Raymondville where Dr. Bennack practiced. That would imply that he had applied for credentials to practice at that hospital. The letter states that since it had been years, 21 to be exact, since his training, there was little information on his record. They did note in the record that his personnel card indicated his "service had been excellent." They apologized for not having more information.

Dr. Bennack had been married prior to medical school and was older than the other medical students because, after attending Pleasantan High School, he worked as a master machinist for the railroad, helping his two younger brothers through dental school. They, in turn, helped him through university and medical school. He had one son while in his first year in medical school. Following his internship, he returned to Raymondville, in South Texas, the town of his birth in 1900, where he practiced until retirement.

Dr. Bennack's son, Gene, born during his first year in medical school, became an orthopedic surgeon. He had two other sons. "Bud" was a farmer who also ran a crop dusting business and was the pilot. The third son, Marvin, became a dentist like his uncles. The orthopedic surgeon and the dentist sons were retired at the time of the interview in 1991 when Dr. Bennack was in his 90's. [5].

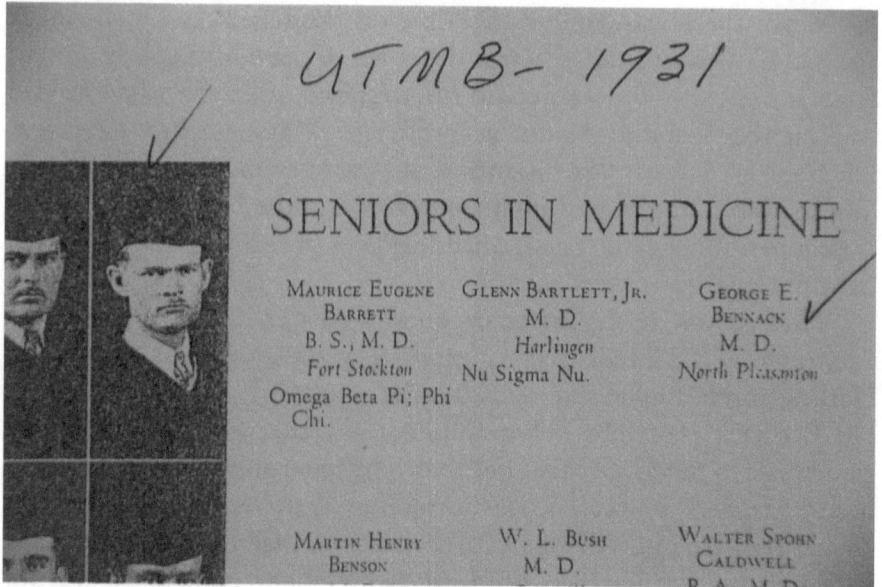

UTMB 1931 graduation picture Dr. George E. Bennack, M.D.

Dr. Claud Martin

The following year, 1932, Brackenridge took on their second trainee. Dr. Claud Martin, M. D. was a classmate of Dr. Bennack but did his internship in Galveston at the John Sealy Hospital, the teaching hospital for the medical school. In medical school, he had been the president of the senior class and was the editor of the yearbook, the "Medical Section Cactus." Having completed his internship at Galveston and then spending most of his time in Austin doing surgical cases, his year would have been considered a residency.

During his training in 1932, he managed to get the hospital to purchase a microscope, a centrifuge and an incubator and water bath that allowed them to set up a lab down the hall from surgery. Prior to that, Dr. Manny Graham came from his office in town to do routine cultures and blood cultures. Although most doctors read their own x-rays, Dr. Horace Gilbert would come to the hospital to read some of the films.

Dr. Fred Lowry, an orthopedic surgeon who came to Austin in 1946, related a story told about Dr. Martin when he was doing his training in Austin. A patient was admitted to the emergency room and, as part of his work up, was sent for a chest x-ray. Dr. Martin went to the radiology department and was there when the patient had a cardiac arrest on the x-ray table. Dr. Martin climbed on the table and started resuscitation with help from the technician. That was unsuccessful and the patient died. The family was there for this activity. When Dr. Martin climbed down to console the family, one of the family members said, "Oh Lordy, you sure can kill 'em quick," obviously completely misunderstanding what was going on.

The operating rooms were on the third floor at the north end of the building. That would have been the Fifteenth Street end of the building. On that same floor, on the south end and toward the back of the building, was the x-ray department and the laboratory. Down the hall, over the area of the front door, was a room for Bertha Spaeth, the operating room supervisor. She lived in that space as well. The patient rooms were on the second floor while the emergency room and clinics were on the first floor toward the back or west side of the building. The main entrance and the administrative offices were on the front of the building facing east toward East Avenue.

Following Dr. Martin's training, he entered private practice in Austin in general medicine and surgery. A few years after starting his practice he did an appendectomy on Lyndon Johnson, by far his most famous patient. It is noted in Lyndon Johnson's biography that he collapsed with appendicitis in the spring of 1937, at the age of 28, while campaigning for Congress as an ardent Roosevelt supporter. This was two days before the election. He learned from his hospital bed that he had won his seat. Dr. Martin continued to practice in Austin until the 1970's, although by that time he was just doing general medicine and not surgery. It is noted in the book "Admissions, The Extraordinary History of Brackenridge Hospital" that Dr. Martin was the nephew of a former city physician.[3]

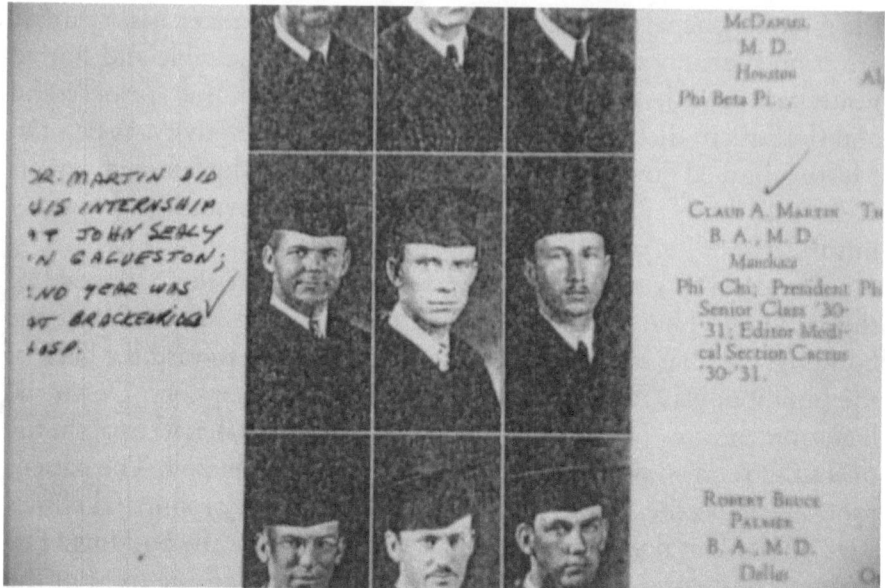

UTMB 1931 graduation picture Dr. Claud A. Martin, M.D.

The election of Lyndon Johnson in 1937 was for his seat as a United States Congressman. This is not the famous 1948 election in which it is said that some names from gravestones were borrowed to help him win. The 1937 election has its twists relative to Austin. Congressman James P. Buchannan, who was involved in obtaining funding for the dam near Burnet, and after whom the dam was named, died suddenly in 1937. Lyndon Johnson decided he wanted to run for the unexpired term. He consulted with an Austin lawyer, Alvin Wirtz, about his chances and was not encouraged. He persisted and became somewhat of a stand out as a staunch Roosevelt supporter. Wirtz and others came around to the idea that Johnson had a chance and would be a strong supporter of continuing federal money for the Marshall Ford Dam, (later the Mansfield Dam) under construction. If the dam was not funded, the project would collapse and the builder, George Brown of Brown and Root, Mr. Wirtz's client, might go bankrupt. He and others threw their support to Lyndon Johnson and he was elected. Of course, the dam was completed under the Lower Colorado River Authority and the U. S. Bureau of Reclamation.

There was no intern listed for the year 1934 and then in 1935 to 1936 Dr. David L. White did his internship. He did not stay in Austin to practice.

The next trainee at Brackenridge was Dr. Charles B. Dildy, M.D., who graduated in 1935 from Baylor University College of Medicine in Dallas. He interned at Emanuel Hospital in Portland, Oregon and then came to Brackenridge for further training before going into general practice in Austin. He was followed by Dr. Tilman E. Dodd, also a graduate of Baylor, who did his internship at Brackenridge before going to John Hopkins Hospital in Baltimore, Maryland. He returned to Austin to practice general medicine and pediatrics.

Medicine in the 1930's

The first orthopaedic surgeon in town, Dr. Sandy Esquivel, came to Austin in 1935. He was born in El Paso, Texas and attended the University of Texas at Austin for his college years. At the university he was the captain of the track team and the basketball team in 1926, set a two mile run record that stood until 1949, was on the 1924 and 1925 Southwest Conference championship track team. He also managed to get grades that took him to medical school at Galveston. Following medical school he interned in Galveston, spent a year at Scott and White in Temple, and then attended the Columbia Presbyterian Hospital, Orthopaedic Surgery residence program. In 1935 he returned to Austin to set up his practice. He trained an orderly, Carl Sundberg, to become an orthopaedic technician. Many general practitioners did their own fracture work in those days. With Carl's added experience, they came to depend on him to help set bones or assist them in cast work. That training allowed Carl to assist in the cast room until the 1970's. Dr. Esquivel did all of his hospital work at Brackenridge and contributed to the clinics and took call in the emergency room for trauma. He would have been a great addition to the interns' training with the latest of techniques for fracture care. He also treated orthopedic cases from the University of Texas student health center. In the early days and even as late as the 1970's there was an operating room at the health center where smaller procedures could be done.

Most fracture care involved closed reductions and casting. Fractures of the femur and tibia and many fractures of the upper arm (humerus) were not suitable for simple casting. In those years most were treated in bed with traction to maintain the alignment of the bone. For a tibia or femur fracture, bed rest could involve two to three months before the fracture was "sticky" enough to be put in a cast. For a femur fracture, a cast involved encasing the whole leg and the lower body, a body cast, to provide adequate protection of the fracture. With hip fractures in the elderly, extended bed rest could be fatal. There were only a couple of fixation devices that could be used in some hip fractures, but they were frequently not sufficiently strong to hold the bone. It was not until the early 1950s that the Moore prosthesis was used for some femoral neck fractures as a replacement for the femoral head. Dr. Esquivel would have been exposed to these devices in his residency in New York where much of this progress was being made. The interns would have been involved in the treatment, especially making rounds on the long-term bed patients. Unfortunately, infected hip wounds would have involved many days of dedicated care and dressing changes. There were no antibiotics available at the time except for sulfa that came on the market around 1937.

The practice of medicine in the 1930's was profoundly affected by the Depression. The unemployment rate was around twenty five percent nationally and most could not pay for medical care. Health insurance had been available from the 1850s on a very limited basis. Most policies were purchased to protect against lost time from work. Hospitals were held in such low regard that most people would not choose inpatient care and thus had little chance of incurring this type of expense. They were mostly cared for at home. In the early 1900s, as health care became safer and more reliable, hospitals began to be more popular. In 1929, Baylor University hospital in Dallas, Texas noted that school teachers had great difficulty paying their medical expenses. Baylor began to offer a program in which teachers could pay 50 cents per month to guarantee 21 days of hospital medical services per year, if needed. During the depression, other hospitals began providing pre-paid health plans. In 1939, the American Hospital Association used the term Blue Cross to designate health care plans that met their standards. These plans were eventually merged to create Blue Cross, a non-profit organization. Blue Shield was created gradually, but consolidated in 1946 to pay for doctor's expenses. Blue Cross and Blue Shield merged in 1971.[6]

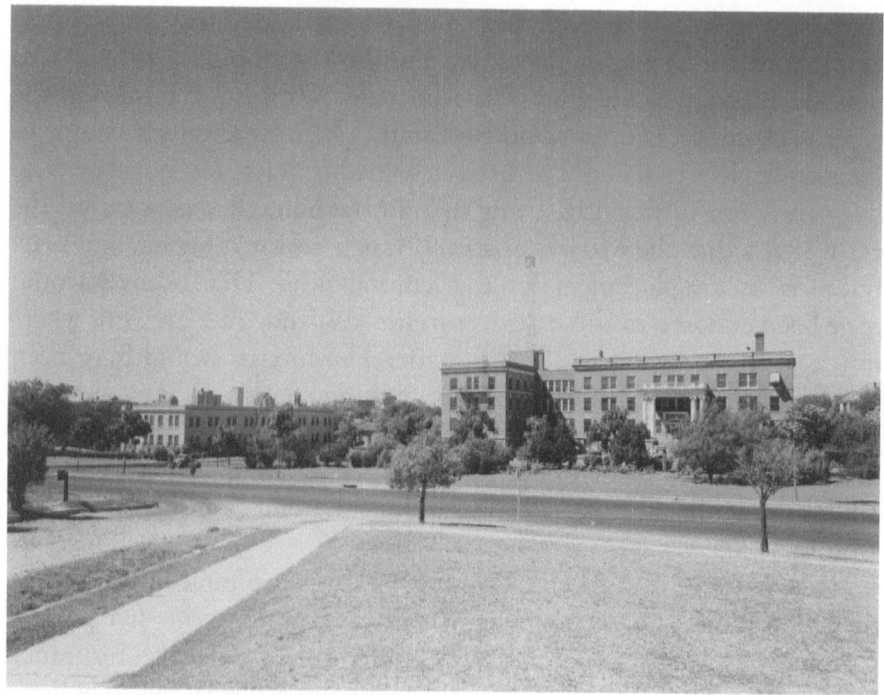

Brackenridge Hospital main building with 1929 south wing addition. School of nursing building to the left (south) of the hospital. (with permission, Austin History Center, Austin Public Library.)

During that period of the 1930's, Mrs. Anita Land, who later worked many years at both Brackenridge and St. David's Hospital, attended nursing school at Brackenridge. The hospital had its own program for nurses training with very little in the way of formal classroom education. It opened in 1915. Eventually a full nursing school was developed, including the nursing building just south of the hospital. During that early time the nursing students learned primarily at the bedside and through their responsibilities working on the floor. The students made up the nursing staff under the supervision of one registered nurse on each unit. The duty hours were from 7 AM to 7 PM or 7 PM to 7 AM. There was a three-hour break in the middle of the day for classes. These were taught by the registered nurses and by doctors from the local community who gave their time for instruction. Mrs. Land noted that they did not worry about overtime as their fellow students came in and took over at the end of the shift.

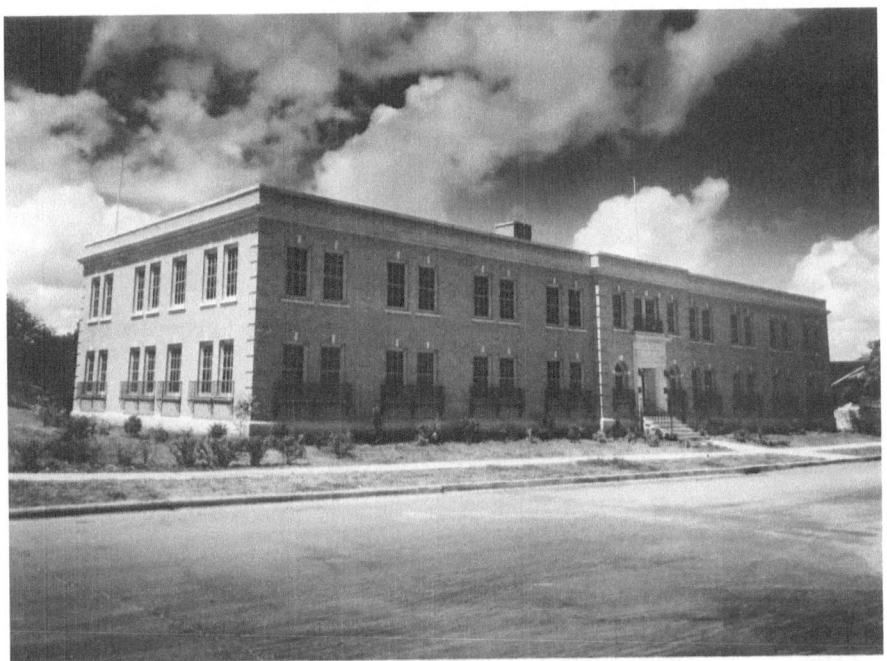

Nursing School building, (with permission, Austin History Center, Austin Public Library.)

Their duties included a daily sponge bath for the patients, provided by the first year students or by a family member, if one was available. There was not always a change of linen but water was never a problem so the bath was a requirement. There were no bathrooms in the patient rooms, but there was a facility down the hall. On each floor there was a hopper room with a faucet and washtub or utility sink. The bedpans were carried down the hall to the hopper room and cleaned. There were not enough bedpans to provide one for each patient so they were cleaned in the hopper room and taken to a different patient after use. Mrs. Land described these as "community utensils." Taking the bedpans to the hopper room was not one of those jobs sought after by the students.

During those years, there were no disposable gloves, needles or syringes. The gloves were washed and hung out to dry after each use. They had to be inspected for holes and the holes were patched. They were then wrapped and sterilized in an autoclave. Syringes were glass. After use, they were taken apart, washed, wrapped and sterilized in the autoclave for the next use. Needles were also washed, sterilized and reused. They would eventually get little hooks on the tips so they would have to be filed sharp before cleaning and reusing.

The hospital was not air conditioned during that time. On hot days the windows were wide open for circulation. The operating room was no exception with windows also open in the summer. During Mrs. Land's training, she recalls that through the open windows one day came the voice of a newspaper boy shouting the news that "Adolf Hitler had invaded Poland." There was a moment of quiet "as the doctors and nurses hesitated in their work to look at each other and voice a prayer for everyone."

There was no labor and delivery suite in the hospital. The expectant mothers stayed in their regular rooms during labor. When they were felt ready to deliver, they were urged onto a stretcher and taken down the hall to the delivery room. Anesthesia was morphine, nitrous oxide or ether.

Segregation was a fact of life and the Negro patients were housed in a separate building. Their early 1900's beds were old and low and had no mechanism for elevating to the level of a stretcher for easy transfer to the delivery room. As a consequence, a number of infants were delivered in the bed, frequently by the nursing student, without the presence of the intern or other doctor. The doctors came later to tie the cord. Doctors Bennack, Martin, Dildy, and Dodd were always on call, as was the full time resident doctor for these duties.

The other duties of the nursing student, besides washing, starching and ironing their dresses, and, of course, their nursing caps, included sweeping and mopping the floors, changing the beds, writing records, giving shots for pain, delivering meals and rubbing backs. A back-rub was just part of the therapy at that time.[7, 8]

The interns participated in patient care in the clinics and the hospital wards. There were limited medications. Sulfonamides became available in 1937 and were found to be very helpful in treating streptococcal throat infections and scarlet fever. Penicillin was not generally available until after World War II. General anesthetics for surgery were provided by morphine, ether, nitrous oxide and chloroform. Nausea was practically universal with ether and treatment was very limited. Aspirin and morphine were available for pain. Insulin was available on a limited basis for diabetes mellitus. The most common surgeries were for trauma, eye injuries, ear infections, and gynecological procedures.

Othere common surgeries included appendectomies, herniorraphies and tonsillectomies.

The interns scrubbed on these cases as time permitted. The most common causes of death were heart disease, cancer and infections with pneumonia, influenza, and syphilis at the top of the list of infections.

Most interns were planning on a general practice and obstetrics was part of that workload. Many practitioners used the rectal rather than a vaginal exam to check the progress of labor and dilation of the cervix. The vaginal exam was considered more accurate though the rectal was safer from a standpoint of infection. Premature rupture of membranes was a very serious concern, as infection could lead to the death of the mother and the child. Rupturing the amnionic membranes or stripping it from the distal uterus were the standard forms of initiating labor. Castor oil, quinine, (intramuscular and intravenous), and petuitrin were chemical means of inducing early labor. The indications for early induction of labor included toxemia (high blood pressure), kidney and cardiac insufficiency, hypertension, and the fear of an oversize baby. Physically measuring the pelvic outlet with instruments or the hand was the standard, as x-rays were not generally used for this purpose. Cesarean sections had been performed well back in history, but infection was a major deterrent. One approach to the procedure involved elevating the peritoneum off the front of the uterus and then closing it to separate the wound from the peritoneal cavity. Slow labor and pelvic dystocia (too large of a head for vaginal delivery) were the primary indications for this risky procedure. As there was no blood bank in Austin until 1951, significant bleeding during pregnancy from placental previa (placenta blocking the cervical opening) and cesarean sections required the staff to find appropriate blood donors before the procedure. ABO typing was initiated in 1908. The first blood bank in the country was at Cook County Hospital in Chicago in 1937.[9, 10, 11]

The EKG, electrocardiograph machine, was developed in 1913 but not available in Austin until Dr. Lang Holland brought one from his office to be used at the hospital in 1939. The machines in those days were relatively small but heavy, came in a wooden box a little larger than a medicine bag, and could be carried to homes and the hospital. Dr. Holland was an energetic man who graduated from Tulane University School of Medicine in 1934, did his internship at Jersey City Medical Center and his residency in medicine at Charity Hospital in

New Orleans. At Brackenridge he either started or participated in the medicine, diabetes mellitus, tuberculosis, and allergy clinics. He held the diabetic clinic on Monday mornings at 7:00 AM so that working people could save a 24-hour urine specimen, bring it to the clinic for testing and still get to work on Mondays relatively early. Brackenridge eventually got an EKG machine of its own. Dr. Holland continued to interpret EKGs and cross-index all the cardiograms taken on staff and private patients until the late 1960's. He apparently donated as much as 40 hours per week at Brackenridge, in additions to his private practice. The interns benefited from his presence in the clinics and his teaching.[12]

Dr. Holland was at the hospital so much that the instructors of the school of nursing would ask him to look at the students when they became ill. This began to happen so often that by 1946 he was given the title of School Physician for the nursing school. He stated that "I get a great deal of pleasure working with the girls and watching them grow from young girls to beautiful young ladies." In 1964, the Executive Committee of Brackenridge Hospital Medical Staff issued a statement of commendation that stated in part that, "Dr. Holland has devoted more time to charity patients than any other doctor in the history of our staff at Brackenridge Hospital. We, therefore, commend him to you as All American Doctor Number 1."[12]

As we look at the training activities at this community hospital in the early years, we might get the impression that this was a unique situation in the country. That is certainly the impression one gets in talking to doctors who have been involved over the years. The numbers would suggest the contrary. Our country and the medical profession appear to have been very dynamic for the one hundred years after the formation of the America Medical Association. Although the guidelines for an internship had been proposed by the AMA 25 year prior, the association was busy approving hospitals for these teaching activities and keeping track of those approved. The recommendations for training programs included having at least 100 hospital beds; a director of education, either part or full time; rotations of at least three months on internal medicine and surgery each, and the training period of one year or longer, as a number of programs were eighteen months. In accrediting hospitals as training facilities, the number of autopsies was considered in the formula. According to the records of the Accreditation Council for Graduate Medical Education contained in "The Green Books," published by the AMA, in 1939 there were 734 hospitals approved for training purposes with slots for 7,833 interns across the country. Many were associated with medical schools but a large number were community hospitals that took on these responsibilities. By 1949, in additions to the internship programs, there were twenty-six specialties recognized with approved residency training programs ranging from Allergy to Urology.[13]

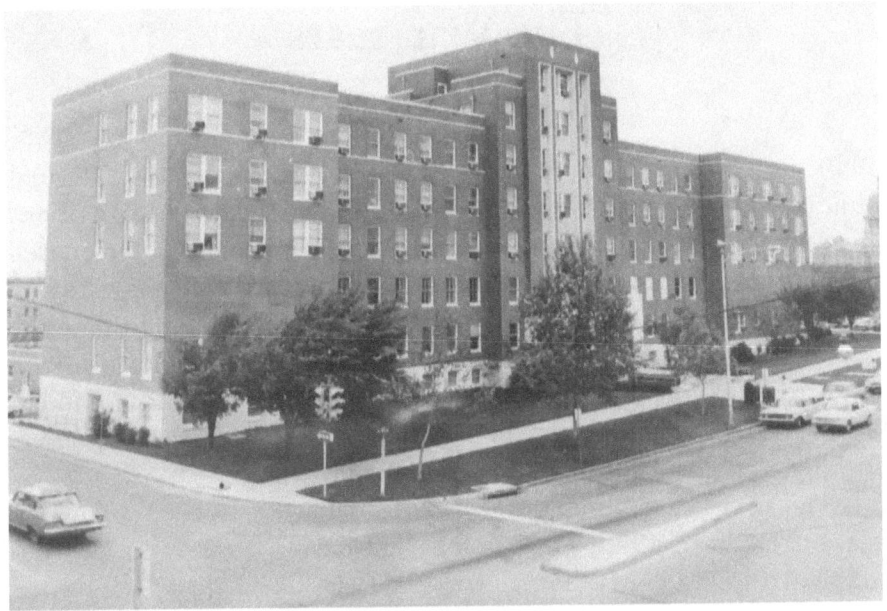

North Wing addition (center tower, 1940) plus east and west extensions (1950s) facing 15th street. . (with permission, Austin History Center, Austin Public Library.

The War Years

1940 was to be a monumental year at Brackenridge. The original building that faced east and fronted on East Avenue had had additions of a south and west wings to provide more space. The west wing housed the negro patients and the south additional beds. Medicine was changing and more patients were admitted as the care was improving. In 1940 the north wing was added. This addition of a seven-story building along 15th Street provided increased beds, bringing the total for the hospital to 209.[3] The top two floors were in a central tower that contained quarters for the interns and additional space for conferences.

The next decade brought Dr. John T. Frawley to the hospital for his internship in 1940. He was followed be Dr. Sam Wilburn, who graduated from UTMB in Galveston in 1941. Dr. Wilburn completed his internship at John Sealy and then came to Brackenridge where he was considered a rotating resident. He was then taken into the Army in 1943 and served as an internist in England and France until 1946. He then completed two years training in Pediatrics at the Children's Medical Center in Dallas, Texas. He returned to Austin in 1948 and practiced pediatrics with twins Lancing and G. Clifford Thorne in an office shared at Medical Arts Square. His time off was spent flying, as he had earned his pilot's license in 1932.[14]

Lancing Thorne completed medical school at the University of Texas Southwestern in Dallas in 1944 and would have been in the first graduating class. Southwestern was created in Dallas after Baylor University College of Medicine moved to Houston in 1943. Dr. Thorne then pursued his internship in Madison Wisconsin followed by a pediatric residency at Texas Children's hospital in Dallas and then Cincinnati Children's. Dr. Clifford Thorne, Dr. Lancing's twin brother, attended medical school at Duke University followed by his pediatric residency in Cincinnati, Ohio. Following the pattern of most doctors who came to Austin, the Thorne brothers established practices at Brackenridge for much of their inpatient work. Their practice included Dr. Willburn in 1948. They each took a month at a time to provide services in the pediatric clinic and were there to supervise the interns and making rounds. In additions, another rotation included covering the Emergency Room, admitting patients that required hospitalization and attending newborn babies in the nursery. Interns would be available for some of these duties under their supervision, but much of the work the community doctors did on their own, including charity care. There were not enough interns to cover all of the services available for patient care. Dr. Wilburn practiced until 2002. That is sixty-one years, if you are counting, from the time of graduation from medical school. He died in Austin in 2006.[14]

The year following Dr. Wilburn, 1942, Dr. Ruth Bain graduated from UTMB, did her internship at St. Louis Hospital in St Louis, Missouri and then came to Brackenridge in 1943, where she completed a year in general practice. Because there was such a shortage of doctors, especially surgeon, during World War II, she completed the rotating internship that evolved into a shortened straight surgical residency at Brackenridge. During WWII approximately one third of practicing doctors were drafted into the military. That created a significant shortage of practicing doctors left in the country. Those remaining doctors were very busy with their offices and the emergency room demands. In 1947 Dr. Bain joined the staff of the University of Texas Student Health Center where she worked until 1953. She then opened a private general practice in 1950 but continued part time service at the Health Center.

A remarkable person, she became involved in the Travis County Medical Society, became the secretary, and in 1962 was the first woman president of the society. She also became involved in the Texas Medical Association, became a member of the Board of Councilors for 10 years and then was elected president of the Texas Medical Association from 1982 to 1983. She was the second woman to have held that position. Not being content with those limited activities she was involved in establishing the Family Practice residency at Brackenridge and between 1974 and 1978 served as Clinical Director, Acting Director and then Associate Director of the program. Thus, having been trained at

Brackenridge, she returned to assist and direct the new training of Family Practice residents in Austin.[15]

The same year that Dr. Bain graduated, 1942, Dr. Otto Brandt, Jr. graduated from UTMB and went to St. Paul Hospital in Dallas for his internship. He then returned to Brackenridge for an additional year of training. As was typical of the time, World War II dominated everyone's schedule. Dr. Brandt was activated into the Army where he served in a Mobile Army Surgical Hospital (MASH) unit in the Philippines. One memorable occasion he related, was giving General McArthur's wife a tour of the facility. At the end of the war he was transferred to Nagasaki, Japan to serve in hospitals there before returning home to start a practice in Austin. He had grown up in Brenham, Texas and later attended the University of Texas, so chose Austin as a practice location. His general practice in Austin lasted fifty-one years, many of those years along side Dr. James Graham, at Medical Park Towers. During those years he delivered many babies at Seton Hospital.

In the late 1940's, there was generally one intern or resident per year. Most were serving one-year internships. Dr. Wilbur Quinten Budd was here in 1946-47; Dr. John H. Cayce, 1947-48; Dr. Sigman W. Hayes, 1948-49; Dr. Benjamin Elliott, 2 years from 1947-49; and Dr. James Richard Sims, 1949-50. Dr. Hayes was the only one of those trainees to remain in Austin to practice. Their training and early practice would have been significantly affected by penicillin that became available to the public after the war. The dose was about 200 mg, aqueous given every six hours or, sometimes, three times per day. I personally recall receiving penicillin in 1948, as a shot in the bottom, administered by our doctor at home on a house call. To limit his number of visits to our house in the country, he taught my mother how to give the shots, which she did for the last several days of the course of treatment. That was, of course, after recovering from her nervousness at my looking back and saying the needle she was using was longer than the doctor's needle.

The later 1940's, after World War II, proved to be active years for the future of postgraduate resident and internship training at Brackenridge. A number of doctors came to town to open practices. Dr. Fred Lowry, Dr. Bert Tisdale (and his wife, Dr. Marie Tisdale, a pediatrician), Dr. Kermit Fox and Dr. Larry Griffin, all orthopaedic surgeons arrived in 1946 through 1948. This improved the coverage of trauma at Brackenridge. There were more new ideas and experience available for the interns. Dr. Fox would be involved in adding a training position in orthopaedics in the 1960s.

During the 1940's and 1950's there was an interesting stabilization in the politics of the City of Austin as Tom Miller was the mayor from 1933 to 1949. He was also the mayor from 1956 to 1961. That is also the period when the hospital was enlarged significantly with the addition of east and west wings to the north section. Dr. Zachery T. Scott was the chief of staff from 1943 to 1946. Rev. John Barclay became a member of the hospital board in 1950 and is listed as a member of the board as late at 1965. He later was a very long time member of the St. David's Board.[3]

A sign of the times found Dr. Marie Tisdale, wife of orthopedist Bert Tisdale, coming to Austin before her husband Bert because of his enlistment during the war.

Although she grew up in Austin, she found opening a pediatric practice full of obstacles. She did her training in Louisiana and under the historic influence of Napoleonic Law there, she obtained her license to practice, could own her own property and conduct her own business. In Texas, as a married woman, all of her property belonged of her husband. As Bert was still in the service, she found she could not lease an office on her own, and the Austin National Bank, where her father had done business for years, was not willing to open an account in her name. Only after some significant work, and perhaps the help of someone who knew her father, was she able to open an account. Fortunately, Dr. Tom McElhenny, another pediatrician in town who was overly busy because so many doctors away in the war, offered her a position to work for him. Note that she "worked for him" but was not offered a partnership arrangement. She felt this was the only way she was going to get started. She accepted the position, and soon became as busy as any doctor in town.[16]

Dr. Bert Tisdale started medical school in Galveston in 1928. The depression started in 1929. On returning to school in 1930 for his third year he was working his way though. He found that he could not continue that. Marie had completed her BA at the University of Texas in 1930. They must have worked for a year or two and then they were married in 1932 without much in the way of money. They both headed off to New Orleans where Marie would start medical school and Bert would enter his third year. Apparently they managed somehow. After graduation, Bert did his orthopedic residency in Shreveport and at

Charity Hospital in New Orleans while Marie finished medical school. They had several years working apart during training and also when Bert was in the service before finally settling in Austin.[16]

Kermit Fox grew up on a farm near Carmine, Texas, speaking only German when he entered school. The grade school he attended was actually built on the corner of his father's farm on land he provided for the purpose. He completed high school in Brenham living with an older sister and started college at Blinn College in Brenham at age 16. He completed his undergraduate education with a year at the University of Texas in Austin and finally attended medical school in Galveston, graduating in 1936. He did a two-year rotating internship in Rochester, New York, because he knew that a lot of the staff had trained at Cornell in New York City. He opened a general practice in Bryan/College Station but was activated into the Army in 1940. He spent his time as the commanding officer at a hospital in Anchorage, Alaska. He was elevated to that position because his experience included running a farm at home, or at least that is the reasoning that his commanding officer gave for his decision. His military experience also included time at Mineral Wells, Texas, and involved being the chief of orthopedic surgery, which was no small matter, as there were 33,000 troops stationed in Mineral Wells. Following discharge he went to the University of Iowa for a year of orthopedic surgery followed by a fellowship at the Campbell Clinic in Memphis, Tennessee. One of his fellow residents, Dr. Larry Griffin, came with him to Austin in 1948 to set up practice. They had the brace-maker at the Campbell Clinic make them some special operating instruments that they brought to Austin. In those days many of the more specialized instruments used in operations were owned by the doctors and not by the hospitals. More amazing was the fact that the administrator of the Campbell Clinic program lent them $3000 to start their practice in Austin.[17]

These tumultuous years of depression, war, and training resulted in many hardships and separations for the families of the doctors who would come to Austin in the 1940's. As many had their education disrupted, perhaps they did not take it so much for granted. This may have been some of the motivation to become involved in the training of younger doctors. These disruptions of schedules by historical events required the training programs to be rather flexible.

In addition to these new orthopedic surgeons coming to town, Dr. W. O. Johnson arrived in 1948 as the first anesthesiologist. He practiced at Brackenridge and must have brought a sigh of relief to the safety of surgery at the time.

Dr. Georgia Felter Legett, who would become one of the pioneers in medical training in Austin, arrived in 1949 with her husband, ophthamologist, Dr. Carey Legett. She had grown up in Austin, attended the University of Texas at Austin, and also the University of Texas Medical Branch in Galveston. She did an internship at Jefferson Davis Hospital in Houston, a two-year program from 1942 to 1944. She then attended a year of obstetrics at the Margaret Hague Maternity Hospital in Jersey City, New Jersey. She had been encouraged to do training there by Dr. Willard Cook at Galveston because they had one of the lowest maternal mortality rates of any hospital in the country. She then did a year of anesthesia at the Philadelphia Lying-In Hospital, where she learned the technique of continuous caudal epidural anesthesia for obstetric patients. (Note that epidural anesthesia for obstetrics was not the common practice in Austin by the anesthesiologists until the late 1970s.) She followed that training with three years of Gynecology at Jersey City Hospital. During that period she spent time with Dr. George Papanicolaou at Cornell Medical School. As he had developed the Papanicolaou cervical smear technique, Dr. Legett was able to bring this useful tool for women's health, the "Pap smear," to Austin.[20] I suspect it was several years before the pathology department became proficient at reading these "Pap Smears," so it may have been some time before they became the useful tool of today.

During her years of training she maintained a friendship with Dr. Willard Cook, the head of Obstetrics at the Medical Branch in Galveston. With his encouragement she developed an interest in a training program. She was involved with the interns at Brackenridge and came in to the hospital to help them with more difficult cases, particularly surgery and potentially complicated deliveries. She was also involved with running the ob./gyn. clinic for indigent patients. She was instrumental in getting local ob./gyn. doctors to work toward a relationship with Dr. Cook's department in Galveston. There is a letter in the file of the Travis County Medical Society from Dr. F. K. Blewett, signed as the chairman of the obstetrics and gynecology department at Brackenridge to Dr. Richard A. Lucas, the chairman of the Intern Resident Committee. In that letter he states, ""I wish to inform you that our department desires to be affiliated with the post-graduate school of medicine of the University of Texas." "Also that we desire (to have) on our service, a one year straight ob. & gyn. resident, also one rotating resident." In that letter he expressed a desire to have an intern on obstetrics and a separate intern on gynecology. It does not appear that there were enough interns to provide all of those services.

Dr. Jimmy Harrod was a practicing obstetrician/gynecologist in the community. He was interested in pathology and ran the tumor and pathology conference for that section and the training program. Dr. Leggett stated that he was well organized and held his conferences regularly each week. It appears that this department was active and progressive in providing services for patients and actively including interns, and later residents, in the program.

In the records at the medical society there is a list of active general practice doctors and obstetrician/gynecologists in the department including Drs. F.A. White, Nelson Shiller, A. H. Neighbors, Jr., H.L. Robinson, McCauley, Scott McGuire, E. K. Blewett, G. W. Cleveland, Samuel Todaro, B. O. White and John D. Weaver.

The Growth Years of the 1950's and 60's

In 1953, after some discussion between Dr. Legett, Dr. Blewett, and Dr. Willard Cook, a program was set up to have OB/GYN residents from Galveston rotate to Austin for part of their training. The first resident was Dr. Frank J. Lee. In 1955 there were four Obstetrics student externs; Leroy Boriack, Charles Hartel, James B. Allison, and Charles Sevens. The resident was Dr. Joseph Durso. Dr. Durso is also pictured in the class of 1954-55 photograph that is on the wall of the training center offices. This was, therefore, the first formal relationship for training with the University of Texas Medical Branch and preceded by fifty years the arrangement to run the several training programs by UTMB in the early 2000's. As Dr. Legett's involvement with Brackenridge centered around helping in the clinics and dealing with the more difficult labor and delivery cases, it is not surprising that a number of her patients were classified as indigent. She remained active until an unfortunate comment by Mr. William Brown, the hospital administrator, questioned the financial solvency of many of the patients classified as Dr. Leggett's patients. They were actually clinic or acute care patients on the obstetric/gynecology service. As this situation was indelicately handled, Dr. Legett felt her services were no longer required at Brackenridge and she admitted further patients to St. David's Hospital as of 1971 after over 20 years of service. According to the records, it would appear that Mr. William Brown became the administrator in 1971. I suspect his reaction to the patient's financial status was influenced by the fact that he was new on the job. Since he was new, it would not be surprising that he would not understand the intricacies of patient admissions of clinic versus private patients. In addition, it would not be surprising that he would want to impress the City with his industry in improving collections for admissions. Thus the purposes of the administrator could clearly be at odds with the purposes of the medical staff.[18]

A letter in my file dated September 4, 2007, from Dr. Legett states that "one of the two greatest honors ever bestowed upon me was the Hall of Fame for Graduate Medical Education in Austin, Texas." She and others were congratulated at a ceremony on June 12, 2007 for their contribution to the program. The ceremony was sponsored by the Seton Family of Hospitals, the Travis County Medical Society, and the University of Texas Medical Branch-Austin Programs. (UTMB was administering the training programs at the time.) It was my pleasure to have been one of the presenters of that recognition because I had been involved with the Travis County Medical Society. Included among the honorees were Drs. B Matt Blackstock, S. H. (Bud) Dryden, George Edwards, David Harshaw, Tom Kirksey, James Lindsey, Earl Matthews, Hector Morales, Robert Pape, Raleigh Ross and Karen Teel.[19]

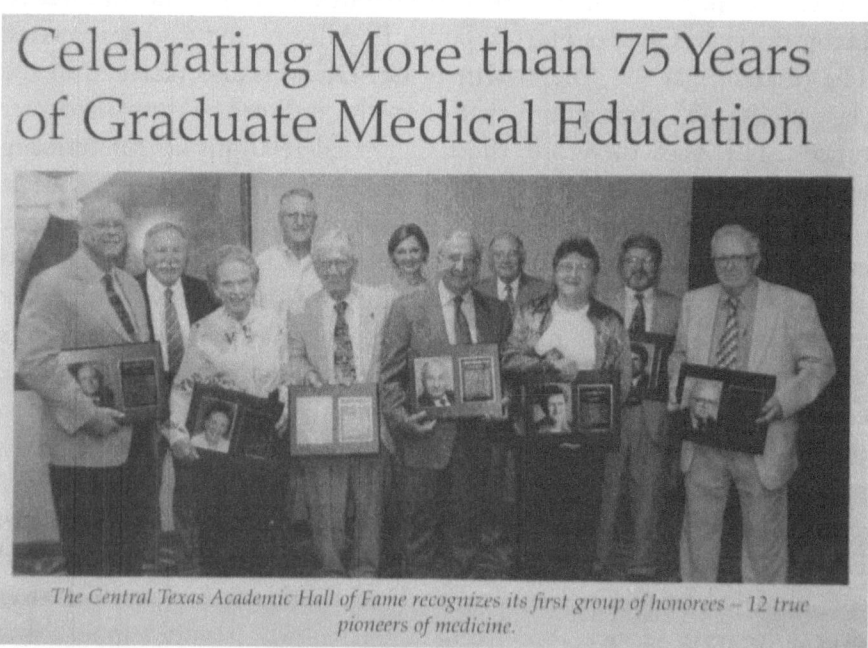

The Central Texas Academic Hall of Fame recognizes its first group of honorees – 12 true pioneers of medicine.

Pioneers of Austin medicine honorees 2007 ceremony (Left to right front: Dr. James Lindsey, Dr. Tom Kirksey, Dr. Georgia Legett, Dr. Mathus Blackstock, Dr. Hector Morales, Dr. Karen Teel, Dr. David Harshaw; back: representatives of the families of Dr. Raleigh Ross and Dr. Bud Dryden, then Dr. Bob Pape and Dr. Earl Matthews.

Dr. Bud Dryden and Dr. Raleigh Ross came to Austin in the late 1940's, and both would make significant contributions to the training program. Dr. S. H. (Bud) Dryden arrived in Austin in 1946, directly out of the army. He was born in Abilene, Texas in 1914, to a father who made tombstones and a mother who had tuberculosis. The family had very little money but he managed to complete his degrees at Abilene Christian College and Baylor University College of Medicine, graduating from Baylor in 1940. He completed an internship at Inter-City Hospital (later Peter Smith Hospital) in Fort Worth to be followed by his induction into the Army Air Corps as a flight surgeon. He was on his way to the Pacific when Pearl Harbor was attacked. He was quickly rerouted to North Africa and field hospital activity in Sicily, Italy, and France. Although he said he felt like he spent most of his time picking up bodies in the field, his hospital experience must have been extensive in both general medicine and surgery. With this background, he settled in Austin with a practice in general medicine and surgery. He delivered many babies and also did a significant amount of orthopedic and general surgery.

When he came to Austin he joined the practice of Dr. Zachary T. Scott and Dr. A. J. (Happy) Scott in an office at Eighth and Brazos. Zachary soon retired and Bud and Happy moved their office to 1303 Sabine, immediately south of Brackenridge Hospital. There were several factors that would shape Dr. Dryden's practice. His humble beginnings led him to treat all types of patients. That background also resulted in a very colorful vocabulary, as he sprinkled his conversation with an interesting array of expletives. He was definitely from the paternalistic era of medicine. He was the doctor and the patients were definitely patients, and there would be no crossing that line. The location of his office on Sabine was just south of the Brackenridge Nursing School building and just steps from the emergency room on the south side of the red brick hospital. Dr. Dryden was very willing to see patients there and developed much of his practice from ER patients. Because of his proximity to the emergency room he started treating many of the policemen who came there for treatment. As a consequence he treated many members of the police force in Austin. His daughter, Jane, describes sitting on a stool next to the nurse's station many hours while he was taking care of patients. Since he did a lot of fracture work, he worked with Carl Sundberg in the cast room. He continued to follow his patients even when they needed another specialist. He would scrub with Dr. Albert Lalonde, a neurosurgeon, when one of his patients needed that care. He did many general surgery and orthopedic surgery cases and would scrub in as assistant when one of his patients was under the care of another surgeon. Dr. Dryden and Dr. Raleigh Ross, a general surgeon, worked together on a number of patients and projects. His practice included a number of East Austin residents, many workers compensation cases, and just anyone who came into his office or the emergency room.

Dr. Dryden was always interested in teaching and he formed a good relationship with the residents and interns. The interns would see a lot of his patients in the emergency room and would follow them in the hospital when admitted. The interns would in many cases act as the primary doctor for patients of Dr. Dryden or one of the other staff doctors. He would give lectures to the interns about various medical and surgical subjects as part of their didactic learning.[20]

Dr. Dryden, along with Dr. John Garcia and Dr. Sam Tadero, would invite the interns out to dinner and, on occasion, invite them over to their homes for a meal. This provided a break to the interns from their busy schedules and rather limited social calendar. Dr. Clinton Cravens, recalls that as an intern, he visited Dr. Dryden's home a couple of times. That tradition was continued into the 1960's when Dr. Cravens was an intern.[21]

The ambulance service in Austin in the early years was supplied by the funeral homes. If a patient needed to be transported, a call was made to one of the funeral homes on a rotating basis. The vehicle for conveyance was the hearse used by the funeral home. There were, of course, no provisions for resuscitation, medications, or other support services except for any first aid that the funeral home personnel might provide. As late as 1966, the Hyltin Manor funeral home, on the service road of IH-35, was called to transport patients from the University of Texas campus during the Charles Whitman shooting from the tower. Morris Hohmann was the driver of one of the ambulances. After transporting one victim to Brackenridge, he was wounded in the leg trying to transport other victims. This serious and chaotic situation was one of the events that would spur the community in the future to commit to providing the dedicated ambulance and emergency services to Austin.[3]

Dr. Dryden, partially because of the vision of pushing for an ambulance service, ran for and was elected to the Austin City Council in 1969. He remained in office until 1973. It was during that time that plans were made to create an emergency medical service.³

Dr. Raleigh Ross, who came to Austin in 1949, would work frequently with Dr. Dryden on projects involving the training program and other issues at Brackenridge. He was born in 1913 in Lockhart, Texas. After graduating from the the University of Texas Medical Branch in 1935, he did his internship and a general surgery residence at the Hospital of Protestant Episcopal Church in Philadelphia. Following that training he was inducted into the Army Medical Corps and served until the end of the war. He did training in general and thoracic surgery that he completed in 1949. He came to Austin were he worked primarily at Brackenridge and, very early on, became interested in advancing the training program in a effort to try to lure good doctors to the community. As part of that effort he was instrumental in obtaining accreditation for the training program under rules of the American Medical Association, the accrediting organization of the time. It is noted that Brackenridge entered the National Residency Matching Plan in July 1953, primarily as the result of Dr. Ross' and Dr. Dryden's efforts.[13]

Dr. Ross formed a partnership with Dr. Murphy Nelson but also worked with Dr. Joe Thorne Gilbert and Dr. John Thomas, all general surgeons. He also had a contract with the Austin State Hospital for surgical care of those patients. Dr. Ross was indeed a go-getter as the records indicated he became chief of the medical staff in 1950, a year or so after coming to Austin.³

Throughout the 1950's and 1960's, he maintained a large surgical practice primarily at Brackenridge. His patients were seen by the interns and the interns also scrubbed on his cases. He participated in the lectures given to the interns. In 1963, in an effort to conform to the rules of the AMA and to better organize the training program, it was decided to hire a doctor to run the training program. Dr. Dryden, as the Chief of the Medical Staff, and Dr. Ross started that process.

The training program had grown a great deal in the twenty years of the 1930's and 40's. In 1951 there were seven interns, two medicine-pediatric residents, a chief surgical resident, and another surgical resident. In 1952 there were seven interns and five residents, including

Dr. Villareal doing his second year in surgery. In 1953 the class consisted of four interns, including Dr. Martin Leggett and Dr. Gerald Senter. Dr. Martin P. Leggett went into practice in Austin. He developed a busy practice partly because he did not make appointments and saw patients on a walk-in basis. His office was on the corner of IH 35 and 32nd street, three doors away from our office, the Austin Bone and Joint Clinic. He would refer a patient to our office almost daily for orthopedic care. A couple of years later he completely stopped referring patients. My partner saw him at lunch one day as asked whether there had been a problem causing him to stop referring to us. He responded that there was a new orthopedic doctor, Dr. Gary Pamplin, who had just come to town. He decided that he would help him get his practice going with frequent referrals. That seemed like a generous thing to do. It must have worked because Dr. Pamplin developed a nice practice. Within a few years, perhaps because we were so close geographically, Dr. Leggett was again sending us patients regularly. Dr. Jerald A. Senter stayed in Austin and developed his general practice. He was very interested in sports and became the team doctor for several high schools.

By 1949 Brackenridge, according to the ACGME records in the AMA report, had 237 beds and 6903 admissions with six internship positions available. At that point, Brackenridge offered $60 per months for internship pay as compared to $25 at Galveston, $20 at Herman, $50 at Methodist, and $75 at St. Josephs Hospitals, all in Houston. The range nationally was $20 to $200 per month. There were a number of Texas cities where positions were offered for internships including El Paso City/County, Harris in Ft. Worth, and Wichita Falls Clinic Hospital.[13]

1954 was a real growth year with ten interns and six residents including three in general practice and one each in pediatrics, surgery, and obstetrics/gynecology. The Ob/Gyn resident, Dr. Joseph Durso was probably one of the residents that Dr. Leggett had arranged to have come from Galveston. The records note, as specifically remembered by Mary Mika, that Dr. Ted Forsythe, an intern, married the chief obstetrical nurse and they moved to Lubbock after completing his year.[5] In 1955 there were fourteen interns and residents. There were eleven interns in the class but there were also four obstetrics externs (students) from the Galveston program, two obstetrics and gynecology residents, and a chief surgery resident.

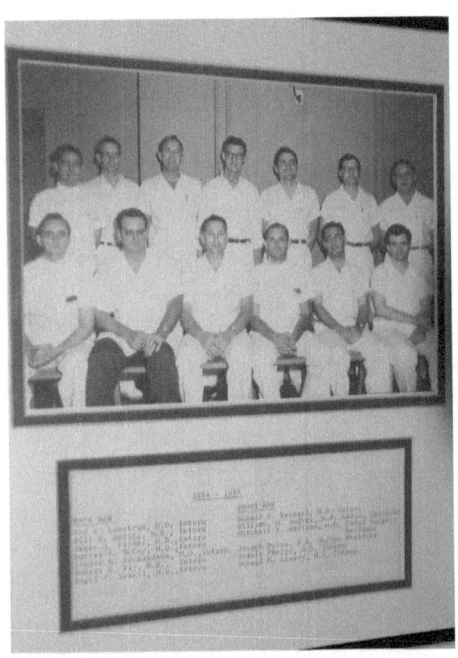

Class of 1954 – 1955 includes Dr. Durso, the first ob./gyn. resident from Galveston.

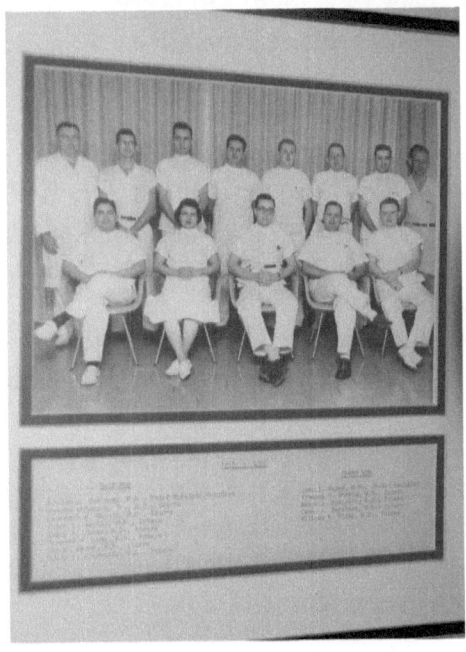

Class of 1955 – 1956.

The class of 1957 included thirteen interns and three ob./gyn. residents from Galveston. In the intern class were Dr. Thomas H. Barnett, Dr. Robert Pape, Dr. Robert Rapp, Dr. Ted M. Sousares, and Dr. V. C Smart, all of whom stayed in Austin for long practices. Dr. Robert Pape played a major role in the training program starting in the 1963. Dr. V. C. Smart did general practice for years in Austin. He decided to get more post-graduate training in Allergy and then returned to Austin for the remainder of his practice in allergy medicine. In 1958 there were thirteen interns including Dr. Francis E. McIntyre who, on completion of his training, opened his general medical practice in Austin. There were also two residents from the Galveston program.

The large majority of trainees were from various Texas cities but the class entering in 1957 included one from Oklahoma and one from New Mexico. That year there were thirteen interns and two residents from Galveston. There were fifteen interns in 1958 with one from Florida, one from Minnesota and the rest from Texas. That class included Dr. Earl F. Grant, who said that he and eight friends from Galveston came to the program. Several of them rented a house in South Austin in which they lived. During their year they rotated through medicine, pediatrics, ob./gyn. and surgery with time on other services and a month in the emergency room. They took night call every third night on the service to which they were assigned and generally had an additional obstetrics night call. Dr. Raleigh Ross and Dr. Swarengen were regularly teachers. Also providing a lot of the teaching were Drs. Fred Lowrey and Kermit Fox in orthopedics; Drs. Marion Stahl, Jimmy Harrod, and Georgia Leggett in obstetrics; Dr. Bud Dryden and Dr. Ruth Bain in general practice. Since most of the pediatricians in town admitted their patients to Brackenridge most of them contributed. The early pediatricians included Drs. Clifford and Lancing Thorne, Sam Wilburn, Ralph Hanna, and William Kelton. The interns admitted many of their patients and the community doctors ran weekly conferences.[22]

In addition to the weekly conferences, as noted above, Drs. Dan Queen, Sidney Bohls, John Rainey, and Charles F. Pelphrey ran the pathology department and held pathology conferences for the interns and residents, starting in the 1950's. Dr. Herrod continued the obstetrics pathology instruction. The pathologists were instrumental in starting a pathology residency-training program in 1955.

Dr. Earl Grant stayed in Austin following his internship and joined the practice of Dr. Jerry Senter and Dr. B. J. Smith. He practiced in Austin for six year before starting a residency in anesthesia at Parkland Hospital in Dallas. He then returned to Austin to join Dr. W. O. Johnson, Dr. Jim Lassiter, and Dr. Earl Yeakel, who did most of their work at Brackenridge before moving their practice to St. David's in the 1970's.[22]

The class starting in 1959 was smaller with only seven interns. That class included Dr. D. A. Baggett who remained in Austin for many years of practice. In that class also was Dr. Abe Rodriguez who went to Barnes Hospital in St. Louis to do an obstetrics/gynecology residence before returning to Austin for his practice. The numbers of interns in each class varied, presumably because the program was not well known outside of Texas and there were only three Texas medical schools at the time, namely UTMB Galveston, Baylor University College of Medicine in Houston, and UT Southwestern in Dallas.

In 1960, fourteen interns started the program. In that class was Dr. Milton J. Railey who stayed in Austin to practice. There were two residents in that year, with Dr. Anthony N. Manoli as a second year resident, having transferred from Metropolitan hospital in New York. He is listed again as a third year resident the next year, 1962. Dr. Norman Anderson is listed as a third year resident in 1960.

The class of 1961 included nine interns, among whom was Dr. Jimmie R. Clemons, who completed his year and then was drafted into the military to serve two years in Viet Nam. In 1975 he returned to Austin after his psychiatry residency to worked at the Austin State Mental Hospital and served on a number of State Commissions. He also accepted responsibilities at Baylor Medical Center in Dallas and, ultimately, was selected as a Distinguished Fellow of the American Psychiatric Association. He retired in 2003 and died in 2005.

Also in 1961 was a husband and wife team, both intern, Drs. Betty and Ross A. McElroy. There were three residents, including Dr. William Risk as a first year, Dr. Pape as a first year surgery resident and Dr. Manoli as a third year. During that period, many of the same community doctors were providing training in surgery, medicine, pediatrics and obstetrics. Dr. Raleigh Ross was scheduling the rotations and Dr. Atys De Silva organized and ran pathology conferences.

A new and important member of the medical community came to Austin in 1958. Dr. R. Maurice Hood contributed several innovations that would affect the medical community in general and the training program specifically. He was not directly involved in the training program but his contributions would change the experience provided in patient care. He was born and raised in Lubbock, Texas by a father who worked in a grocery store but later became a full time fireman. Dr. Hood attended Texas Tech University in 1941 where the tuition was $25 per semester and he could save money by living at home. He joined the Naval Reserve V-1 program that was for pre-medical students. This resulted in an accelerated two-year college program before entering Baylor College of Medicine in 1943. Baylor was part of Baylor University in Waco and was not well funded by the regents. The Southwestern Medical Foundation had been formed to provide additional funds to upgrade the medical school. Baylor, however, was offered a significant amount of money by the M. D. Anderson Foundation to join the new Texas Medical Center in Houston. With additional money from Roy and Lillie Cullen, who built the first building, the medical school moved to Houston in 1943. This left the Southwestern Foundation scrambling to replace the medical school in Dallas. Many of the students and about 90% of the faculty remained in Dallas where classes were held in a junior high school, a converted auto repair garage, other temporary buildings, Parkland Hospital and other local hospitals. It is interesting that these two medical schools, both of which would become pre-eminent teaching institutions, had their new starts in 1943 in temporary buildings, Baylor in Sears warehouse buildings in Houston and Southwestern partially in an auto garage in Dallas.

Meanwhile, Dr. Hood continued his classes and clinical work in Dallas and, again, because of the war, graduated in 1946 from a three-year program. He did an internship at Baylor Hospital and then served in the Navy for eleven years that included his thoracic surgery training. He had enormous experience in chest diseases and surgery. When he came to Austin in 1958 he began a program of cardiovascular and thoracic surgery at Brackenridge. In the early 1960s, as part of the introduction of Austin to open heart surgery and transplant procedures, he, along with Dr. James Lassiter (anesthesiology), Dr. Robert Farris (neurosurgery), and Dr. Walter D. Roberts (internal medicine) convinced the administration in 1960 to convert three south, in the older part of the red brick building, into a twelve bed intensive care unit (ICU). It functioned well for about a year but was staffed by nurses from the general nursing service. The nurses were not dedicated or assigned specifically to the intensive care unit but rotated in from general patient care on the nursing floors. Under these circumstances, the care deteriorated. Eventually, under the direction of Norma White, R.N., the director of surgery, nurses became specifically assigned to the ICU and the care returned to its former level of the first year. This ICU was only the fourth intensive care unit in Texas at the time. It allowed for the first open heart surgery, most likely the repair of an atrial septal defect, to be completed in August of 1961.[3] Patients with illnesses other than cardiac problems were admitted to the ICU. Some were severely-injured patients from the emergency room, so the interns and residents who followed these patients had exposure to improved monitoring, the use of ventilators, ECG monitors, blood gas studies, and arterial pressure monitoring. That space in the red brick building remained the ICU in use until 1978 when the new hospital was completed. I saw patients in that unit when I arrived in Austin in 1971.

As mentioned earlier, Dr. Hood's father started working in a grocery store and was a volunteer fireman until he became a full time fireman. Dr. Hood spent a lot of time at the fire stations to be close to his father while on duty. This led to a lifelong fascination with the fire department. He had a radio monitor in his car so that he could listen and even respond to fire and emergency calls while living in Austin. Ambulance service before the early 1970's, consisted of the services of the funeral home's hearses to transport patients. The Fire Department was also responding to many emergencies by this time and Dr. Hood spent many hours training firemen for emergency services. The City of Austin was resistant to forming a new ambulance service, in spite of encouragement by Dr. Hood, the fire department, and the Travis County Medical Society. In response to the passage of the Federal Emergency Medical Services Act of 1973 and $185 million in federal development money, the State of Texas introduced laws that established guidelines for Emergency Services in the state, ultimately encouraging the formation of an Emergency Medical Service in Austin. The department was developed as a separate department of Emergency Services, rather the within the fire department. This service was developed in the mid

1970s, paralleling the marked growth in emergency room service and the transformation of the training program, to be described later.[23,24]

During the period from the 1930's through the 1960's the number of doctors in Austin continued to grow and the tradition of caring for indigent, as well as insured or "private pay" patients maintained a good pace. When new doctors came to town they were expected to take their turn rotating in the clinics and covering the emergency room. This also involved admitting patients as necessary. With the growth in population and the increasing number of specialists coming to town, the general medical and specialty clinics also grew. This expanded the experience for teaching interns and residents in all levels of the hospital.

In an effort to be as complete as possible I will indulge in listing as many doctors in the late 1950's and 1960's who were quite active at Brackenridge, because they were the backbone of the training program before the rather dramatic changes that would occur with the formation of the Central Texas Medical Foundation in 1972.

In general medicine and internal medicine there were the older workhorses like Drs. Lang Holland, Ruth Bain, Claud Martin, Otto Brandt, B.O. White, Martin Legett, Seldon Baggett, Bud Dryden, and Mathis Blackstock. To this list were added a number of more recent graduates from Brackenridge including Dr. Jerald Senter, Earl Grant, before he studied anesthesiology, V. C. Smart, D. A. Baggett, Milton Railey, France McIntyre, and L. E. Arnold. There was not a separate general practice section at Brackenridge in the early days and the Family Practice designation had not been adopted. The general practitioners mostly attended the surgery and obstetric/gynecology section meetings to make sure they were represented on those services specifically, and on the medical staff in general.

The internists included Drs. Virgil Lawlis, Homer Goehrs, Leonard Sayers, and a little later Dr. Henry Renfert who arrived in the 1950s. These were the founding members of the Austin Diagnostic Clinic that would grow to a large multispecialty clinic in the future. Practicing together, several internists including Charles Darnell, Horace Cromer and Frank Pearce had varying involvement at Brackenridge. Thomas Runge, Walter Sjoberg, and later Stanley Glazener and Homer Goehrs arrived. The interns and residents would evaluate patients in the emergency room and make admissions as necessary to the services of either the general practitioners or internists who were on call, including those listed above.

In the surgery department were Raleigh Ross, Sam Swerington, Murphy Nelson, Joe Thorne Gilbert, John Thomas, Matt Kreisle, Richard Lucas, Will Watt, Ed Zidd, and Ben Simms. The surgery section included the thoracic and vascular surgeons Drs. Maurice Hood, Jimmy Calhoon, Homer (Hap) Arnold, Tom Kirksey, and Bob Tate. Surgery in addition to medicine, pediatrics and obstetric. was one of the primary services through which the interns rotated. The interns spent many hours in surgery, the emergency room, and on the floors taking care of those patients who had been admitted and were mentored by the staff doctors. Regular conferences were also conducted for further instruction, although they were not as well coordinated as would be the case in later years.

The obstetricians and gynecologists providing services were Georgia Legett, James Herrod, Joe Lancaster, Truman Morris, Milton Turner, Fred Hansen and Joe McIlhaney. They took call for the emergency room consultations, admitted patients with the residents, came in for complicated problems or whenever the residents needed help, and ran the service on a rotating basis. It appears that Georgia Legett came in for most of the complicated obstetrics cases for the residents in the 1950's and 1960's.

The pediatric department consisted of a remarkably loyal group of doctors who admitted most of their patients to Brackenridge. Those included Drs. Sam Wilborn, and Clifford and Lansing Thorne who have been mentioned before. In addition, Drs. James Coleman, Clift Price, Miles Sedberry, Pat Cato, Maurice Cohn, Ralph Hanna, Thomas McEllhanney, Gretchen Runge, William Holden, and Ben White were very active. They regularly had interns on their service who were also involved in the delivery room. They covered clinics and emergency admissions. The pediatricians provided lectures regularly, rotating through various topics.

The earliest two neurosurgeons were Dr. Albert LaLonde and Dr. Bob Farris. Drs. Marvin Cressman and Bill Turpin came in the 1960's and were involved in the implementation of the intensive care unit that was so important for brain trauma from the emergency room and surgeries to the brain.

A major tragedy occurred in 1969 that profoundly affected the medical community and particularly the neurosurgery department. Dr. Bob Farris was a pilot and planned on attending a neurosurgical meeting in Washington D.C. in April of that year. He knew a student at Galveston who was interested in neurosurgery, who he wanted to encourage, and who had prepared a paper to be presented to the meeting in Washington. Dr. Ferris, his wife Charlotte, daughters Judy and Maryland, and associate Dr. Ben Becker flew to Galveston, picked up the student Jimmy Dickens, and flew on to Washington, D. C. They then returned to Austin with uneventful stops along the way. On landing at Mueller Airport they were within a few feet of the runway when, perhaps by disturbed air from a passenger jet that landed before them, their plane suddenly lurched up to a hundred feet or so, flipped over and crashed into some houses near the airport. They were all killed, as were two persons in the houses. Jimmy Dickens was a classmate and good friend of Richard Holt, who later became a pediatrician and will be introduced later in this writing. In 1974 a suit was filed by the Dickens family against the federal government and the Federal Aviation Administration regarding the flight control of the two aircraft. Of course, it would not bring any of the victims back.[25]

There were a number of orthopedic surgeons including Drs. Sandy Esquivel, Fred Lowry, Bert Tisdale, Kermit Fox, Larry Griffin, Bob Dennison, Joe Abel, Philip Overton, Elwood Eichler, Tim Lowry, Jerry Julian, and L. Don Greenway who arrived between 1935 and 1970. The general surgeons and orthopedic surgeons were extremely busy in the emergency room and admitted a large number of patients, as the incidence of motor vehicle accidents, gunshot wounds, and other trauma continued to increase. Someone on the staff in 1970 took a count and noted that the general surgeons would be called to the emergency room approximately 110 times per month on average. The orthopedist would get called about 105 times per month. Although the interns and residents seldom admitted the orthopedic patients, they were always involved when there were associated general surgery problems. They also rotated through the specialty clinics of various services. Orthopedics had a cast clinic for fracture follow up appointments and a general orthopedic clinic for back pain, shoulder pain, and more general problems in the follow up of indigent patients. Depending on their interest level, the interns periodically attended these as well. In the period of time from the 1930's to the 1960's, 90% or more of all orthopedics surgical cases in town were done at Brackenridge. They had the only emergency room and the most complete set of orthopedic surgical instruments and hardware, so all major trauma cases were brought to Brackenridge by the various ambulance services.

Neither St. David's, then on 17th Street, nor Seton on 26th street had a dedicated emergency room. The new Seton Hospital was completed on 38th Street in 1975 and included a dedicated ER with a staff. St. David's moved to 32nd Street in 1955 and started with three floors and 52 beds. It had no emergency room. It expanded with a third floor in 1961 and built a fourth and fifth floor by 1968, but still no emergency room. It was not until the early 1980's that they developed an ER with some expansion and remodeling.

The medical community was what might be called "fluid" in the early years. By that I mean that doctors did not limit their hospital practices to one facility but would respond to calls by patients or referring doctors to Brackenridge, St. David's, Seton, and to Holy Cross, a hospital in East Austin. That meant a rather collegial medical community. As a consequence, doctors took emergency room call, clinics, and teaching responsibilities at Brackenridge in addition to their office practice and their services to patients at the other hospitals. That resulted in a rather busy schedule of travel. It is true that some took much more responsibility at Brackenridge and admitted most of their patients there while other concentrated their practices at Seton or St. David's.

Most services or sections, including general surgery, internal medicine, pediatrics, obstetrics and gynecology, orthopedics, urology, ear, nose, and throat, eye, plastic surgery, and psychiatry had regular rotation schedules for community doctors to cover the emergency room and clinics and other responsibilities that were necessary to keep the hospital running. In the early years the general practitioners and a few specialists covered the work schedule. As time progressed into the 1950's and 60's more and more specialists came to town and established more formal sections with regular call rotations, regular meetings, conferences, and more formal teaching duties. And the hospital was getting much busier. By the early 1970's, the orthopedic call schedule became quite demanding to cover the emergency room and the clinic responsibilities. The tradition had been for one doctor to rotate ER coverage for a month at a time. During that month, as the workload increased, it became much more difficult to manage that duty while maintaining a private office practice. The orthopedic section, therefore, found it necessary to spread the work out by changing the call to one night at a time as of 1971. That way they would spend the night covering the ER and the next few days dealing with the injured patients that had been admitted. Frequently surgery was performed on admission and the patient was admitted to the floor for after care. A separate rotation was established so that a different doctor in the section would cover the clinics for a month at a time. These changes made the work load much more manageable.

I have not listed all of the doctors of different services who spent many hours at Brackenridge. The ear, nose and throat, plastic surgery, neurology, gastroenterology, hematology, and many more sections developed services as more and more specialists came to town and more patients showed up at the hospital. As noted earlier, there was an ear, nose and throat clinic as early as the 1930's. I must say, that as the number of doctors increased along with the growth in specialties and sub-specialties, the system became more fragmented. As the other hospitals developed more services, more and more doctors began to limit their practices and many no longer came to Brackenridge as the central medical facility in the community.

A classic example of this evolution involved the cardiovascular surgery section. Cardiovascular surgery started at Brackenridge with Dr. Hood as the only cardiovascular surgeon in town and the only intensive care unit in town. As years passed, the demand for services increased along with the need for space, specialized nursing, surgical equipment, and ancillary facilities. The center of cardiovascular activity moved to St. David's, then to Seton and finally to the Heart Hospital. This evolution and movement revolved around the perceived needs of the doctors, the personalities involved, money, responsiveness of the various facilities, competition between the hospital facilities and the amazing growth of advertising by the hospitals. This evolution was not limited to cardiovascular surgery, but included neurosurgery, orthopedics and, to a lesser extent, the other services. Pediatrics was the first service to actually obtain a separate hospital but rehabilitation hospitals were soon to follow with individual facilities.

Now back to our story of the growth of the training program. The experience of the interns and residents would invariably be influenced by the changes that occurred in the greater medical community and the varying involvement of certain segments of that community at Brackenridge. The popularity of Austin and central Texas as a destination would lead to more and more trainees selecting Brackenridge as a place to gain further experience.

The 1962-63 class of trainees included eleven interns including Drs. Robert S. Alexander, Fred B. Anderson, Henry J. Boehm, Leslie R. Bornfleth, Glenn C. Coates, Clinton E. Craven, Houston G. Hambry, John L. Humphrey, Gary N. Pamplin, Robert A. Tate, and Willis M. Thorstad. Dr. Gary Pamplin completed an orthopedic residency in Colorado and returned to Austin to practice. As noted earlier, Dr. Legget began sending him patients to help him get started. Dr. Bob Tate came with Dr. Craven from the class in Galveston. He was familiar with Austin as he had lived here with his family in the 1940's while his father was stationed at Camp Swift near Bastrop.

Dr. Clinton Craven had gone to medical school in Galveston and during his senior year had done a ten-week preceptorship with a general practitioner in Bastrop. They would refer some of the patients to Austin. That introduced him to Austin as a potential place to do his internship, an idea that he followed. He recalled that during his internship, he rotated through surgery, medicine, pediatrics and obstetrics, anesthesia, and the emergency room, lived on the 7th floor of the hospital, and took most of his meal in the hospital. He noted that the married interns would bring their families to the hospital for many of the evening meals, since it was available and they were always short of money. During his obstetric rotation he was on call 12 hours and then off for 12 hours. He recalled that in pediatrics much of the teaching was done by Dr. Cliff Price, the Thorne brothers, and Dr. Sam Wilborn. Other memorable teachers were D. A. Baggett in general practice, Raleigh Ross in surgery, Bert Tisdale and Kermit Fox in orthopedics and Bob Snider in radiology. Following his internship here, he would complete a pediatric residency at UTMB, Galveston, do his military years stationed at Bergstrom Air Force Base under the Berry Plan, and return to Austin to practice.[21]

Progress in Organization

In 1963, Dr. Robert Pape was in his last year as a resident in general surgery. He had completed an internship at Brackenridge in 1957 and then spent two years at the National Naval Medical Center at Bethesda, assigned to a small project with NASA. He had a masters degree in physiology that qualified him to do studies regarding G-forces that might be encountered by astronauts on re-entry and potential loss of control of the capsules. He then returned to Austin to do a surgery residency. Dr. Raleigh Ross was in charge of scheduling the resident's rotations on the various services and Dr. Bud Dryden was the chief of the medical staff. Dr. Dan Queen, chief of pathology, had taken on the job of part time director of the training program. Dr. Queen then left to become head of pathology at the new Methodist Hospital in San Antonio. His partner, Dr. Atys Da Silva, became the head of pathology and the nominal head of the training program. When in his third year of surgery residency, Dr. Pape was asked if he would consider becoming the associate director of the training program. He would be the assistant to a doctor from New Orleans, who was currently a professor at Louisiana State University Medical School, and who had signed a contract to be the director of training in Austin. The American Medical Association Council on Medical Education stated in 1963 that teaching hospitals would be required to have a full time director of medical education if the program was to be accredited.

Dr. Pape agreed to take on that responsibility. He was born and raised in Seguin, Texas and Austin would be close to home. During his third and last year of residency, he went to New Orleans during Easter break to visit a friend. The friend was an FBI agent transferred to Gulfport, Mississippi because of racial tensions. Dr. Pape read in the

New Orleans Tribune that the doctor who had signed the contract to be the director had suddenly died. On returning to Austin, he informed Dr. Dryden of this serious event. They needed to check out that information and confirm that this was actually the doctor with whom they had the contract. They were at that time a month away from the end of training year in June. After checking, it was confirmed that the doctor had died. As is not surprising, if one remembers Dr. Dryden and his direct blunt approach, he said to Dr. Pape, "We are pretty tight and need someone." He suggested that Dr. Pape take the job for a year or two as an Associate Director of Education while they decided what their next move was to be. As Dr. Pape had made out the call schedules and service schedules rotations for other residents when he was a senior resident, he was at least familiar with that part of the process. He called the medical school in Dallas and arranged a three-day meeting with the director of the residency program at Southwestern Medical School so that, as he said, "I could learn the ropes." Thus, he started his job of Associate Director of Education at Brackenridge, at a salary of $9,900 per year, without finishing his residency. Actually, he did not complete his last year as a resident as he spent the next ten years as medical director. He had even thought of doing an orthopedic or neurosurgery residency but that never happened.

Bob was a very affable person and had a good relationship with the interns, residents, and many of the medical staff. He was also single with no busy family schedule. He, therefore, spent many evenings in the emergency room helping the interns with their patients. In 1966, he was elevated to Medical Director of the program. During those years Dr. Atys Da Silva continued to hold weekly pathology conferences. Dr. Sam Tedaro held Friday breakfast obstetric/gynecology conferences and would also invite trainees to Cosmo's restaurant for a monthly gynecology session. Dr. Joe Rude held weekly review of radiographs and Raleigh Ross held a Saturday surgery conferences and was usually available for Sunday surgery grand rounds. Bob attended all the seminars, clinics and rounds. Dr. Bob Farris, a neurosurgeon, regularly took interns to rotate with him on his service and he and Bud Dryden would fly their planes down to Galveston for recruiting sessions. Many of the surgeons, internists, pediatricians, and other specialists would participate in conferences when the subject was in their area of expertise. They would have to arrange their office schedule ahead of time. Lang

Holland was still reading all the EKGs in those years and this was a great learning tool for the interns. Dr. Tom Runge took over many of Dr. Holland's duties after he came to town. Dr. Albert LaLonde, the first neurosurgeon in town in 1949, and Dr. Robert Farris were very accepting of the interns and Dr. Pape "loved them" for their willingness to be involved. Dr. Farris would fill in as speaker if the scheduled noon speaker for conference had to cancel for some reason. Surgeons, with their cases sometimes going late, were apt to cancel at the last minute.[26]

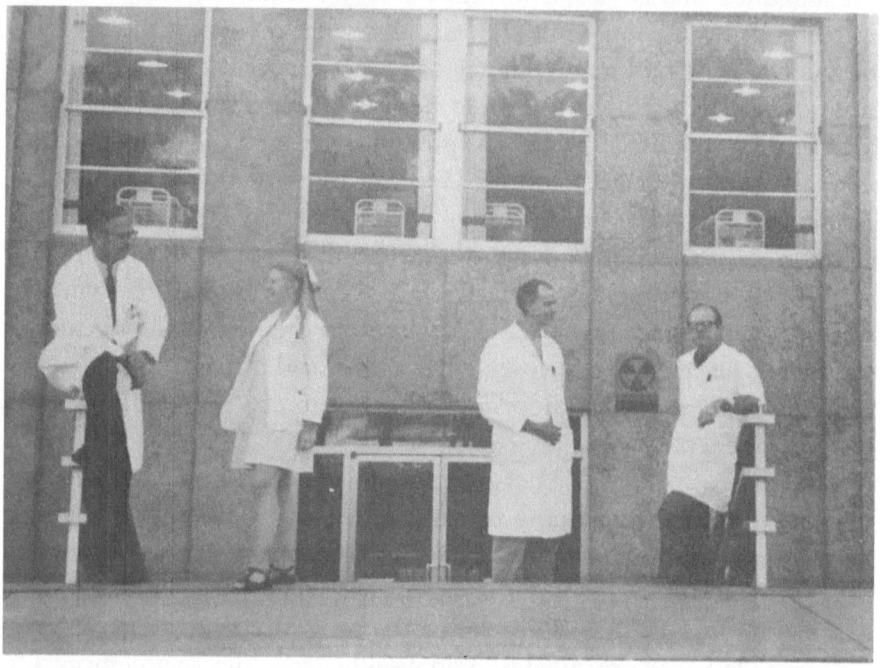

Recruiting brochure for internship program. Dr. Bob Pape on the right.

Between 1965 and 1967, Dr. Kermit Fox worked on a program with Dr. Hanes Brindley, an orthopedist he knew from his training at the Campbell Clinic, in Memphis, Tennesse. Dr. Brindley was then at Scott and White Clinic in Temple, Texas. They arranged to have an orthopedic resident rotated to Brackenridge from that program. The rotations were to be for three to six months. It is always difficult for residents to rotate away from their home program, as arrangements have to be made for living quarters, conferences and supervision. Those problems eventually caused the program to last only two years.

In 1968, Dr. Pape volunteered to be the doctor at a Travis High versus Johnson High School football game. He was knocked down on the sidelines and fractured his tibial plateau. Orthopedist Dr. Bob Dennison operated and elevated the fragment in his tibial plateau and placed him in a long leg case.

Dr. Pape had regularly assisted the residents in surgery but his recovery was complicated by the cast and crutches so he had to stop those activities that required long standing. As a consequence he spent much of the next two years backing up the emergency room interns during the day and spending time in the ER on busy nights.

In 1969 he attended the Congress on Medical Education at the American Medical Association Meeting in Chicago. At the meeting he learned that the Association of American Medical Colleges was no longer going to accredit "free standing" internship programs that had no affiliation with a medical school or with a formal residency training program. In addition, accredited programs would have to have a cadaver available for dissection and would have to meet certain standards for conferences. Starting in 1975, internships of the future were going to have to be integrated into residency programs as a first year rotation. It would also be necessary to have full time supervision of interns in the emergency room, but emergency room rotations for interns would not be mandatory. Much of this was designed to shorten training programs and increase the number of doctors being trained. There were more medical schools being built as well. As a way of increasing the supply of all specialties, it was felt that shortening the post graduate training would help. By compressing the internship into the residency program, a one-year internship and four-year residency could be shortened into a four year program. These changes would profoundly affect the Brackenridge program by ending rotations of interns in the ER, requiring integration of the internship year in other services, and generally requiring much more organization of the training program as a whole. Interns had provided the major work force in the emergency room and the loss of this labor force would result in significant difficulties covering the work load.

It was shortly after that, in 1969, that an affiliation with St. Joseph Hospital in Houston was established for rotations of obstetric and gynecology residents. This would replace the program that had been established with UTMB in the 1950's. In 1970 an arrangement was made for surgery residents to rotate from St. Joseph as well. Putting those doctors on services that rotated regularly in the emergency room would be a help, in addition to their contribution to the patient care inside the hospital.

Dr. Pape was associate director for two years and then was made director. He continued in that role for 10 years, until 1973. In 1972 the Travis County Medical Society was forming the Central Texas Medical Foundation (CTMF) to establish a more formal program. This would result in major changes to the organization of the program and would formalize the various services. To adapt to the AMA rules, directors for the various services would have to be selected.

Dr. Tom Kirksey and Dr. Pape went to Galveston to talk to the head of Pediatrics, Dr. Bill Daeschner, regarding a possible relationship. He suggested that they visit a program in Pensacola, Florida to observe their program. There a community supported residency training program involved the City Hospital, a Catholic hospital and a Baptist hospital was operating. Their training program was organized in a manner that was approved by the AMA. All of these efforts were made to see what the possibilities were to continue the training program in Austin with no medical school and no existing formal residency training. Thus, Dr. Kirksey and Dr. Pape made the trip to Pensacola and spoke with the officials of that program to look at its structure, bylaws, and procedures that might apply in Austin and satisfy the AMA. This would be useful information to provide the Travis County Medical Society in its deliberations for forming a community based program.

Dr. Pape continued to work with the development of the program as the Central Texas Medical Foundation was formed in 1972. He was Medical Director until 1973. He worked in the ER with the interns until they were incorporated into the medicine department. He worked shifts in the ER and was doing so in 1975 when Dr. Don Connell started working there. Dr. Pape then joined the general practice of Dr. Bud Dryden for five years followed by an attempt, with five other doctors, to open an urgent care center that eventually did not work out. He then went into a general practice setting with Dr. Charley Gregory and continued that until retirement in 1994. He, therefore, as the first director of the medical education program, was involved in creating exchange programs in surgery and obstetrics and gynecology with St. Joseph Hospital in Houston, and with improving the internship program with more organized lectures and more regular supervision in the ER as well as worked through the changes in intern ER rotations. He helped bring the ideas of the Pensacola program to Austin, and coordinated the transition of the training program to the next phase, with full time directors of the surgery, medicine, pediatrics, and obstetrics and gynecology sections. He was also quite involved with training of emergency medical technicians (EMTs) in a newly formed emergency medical service.[26]

Coming into the training program in 1963 were ten interns and residents. The five interns were Lt. James R. Finch, Capt. Gary R. Jones, William L. Lemon, Edwin E. Owens and June E Richardson. The residents were Waldo Gonzalez from Mexico, Milton H. Stern, Capt. Lawrence I. Stuart, Herman R. Van Sickle and James Thomas Walker. In this group, Dr. Gary Jones went on to complete an obstetrics/gynecology residency and returned to Austin for his practice. Dr. June Richardson started her general practice in Austin.

In 1964, the interns were Drs. Dana B. Copp, Walter R. Konzen, Fredrick R. Petmecky, Charles E. Strauss, Presley Joe Mock and Richard L. Ballard. Dr. J. Fred Kramer was the chief surgical resident and Dr. Franklin C. Harmon was also a resident. Dr. James L. Spidle started his first year as a pathology resident and Drs. Norman Miles and David Haggard were ob./gyn. residents. Dr. Richard Ballard went on to a pathology residency at Baptist Memorial hospital in San Antonio and returned to Austin to practice.

1965 brought a large class. There were eleven interns including Drs. Travis L. Casler, Howard B. Condren, Herbert Davis, Ralph H. Gay, Vernon Eugene (Gene) Grove, Robert Haxelwood, Richard Orr, Robert Potts, Joe R. Reneau, Samuel H. Shaddock and Richard L. Weddige. Dr. Joe Reneau would remain in Austin for his general practice. Dr. Grove completed a psychiatry residency and returned to Austin for his practice.

The residents for that year included Dr. Fredrick Harmonn as chief surgical resident after his previous year in surgery at Brackenridge. Dr. Robert Tate was a first year surgical resident; Dr. Spidle, second year pathology; and Dr. Sidney Smith, Michael Howard and James Taylor Wharton were Ob/Gyn residents from Galveston.

The class of 1966 included 10 interns. These were Drs. Weldon L. Ash, Michael J. Daughety, Everett M. Donowho, Thomas P. Fagan,

Curtis S Heinrich, F. Howard Hughes, Thomas F. Lowe, Charles M. Myers, Lynn R. Nesbitt, and R. Al Trompler. None of that class stayed in Austin to practice. The residents for that year included Drs. Robert Tate, second year surgery; James Spidle, third year pathology; Francisco Veloz, first year surgery; and Pramool Sukawatana. It is noted in the records, not surprisingly with the large classes, that only Dr. Thomas Fagan is listed as living at Brackenridge. Most of the trainees during the 1960s lived "off campus." There certainly was not room for them to live at the hospital.

The interns for 1967 included Drs. John Baker, Raymond Buck, Jan Howard, Dicky Huey, Bill Schuessler, Alfred Williams, and James Winn. Dr. John Baker returned to UTMB for an obstetrics/gynecology residency and then came back to Austin to join a practice here. The residents were Dr. Tate, third year surgery; Travis Casler, who did his internship in 1965; Dr. Ricky Donowho, first year and Dr. James Spidle fourth year pathology; Francisco Veloz, second year surgery and David Shannon and Gene Jones, residents whose specialty is not listed. Dr. Quiroga was the resident who came from Scott and White Clinic for his orthopedic surgery rotation. He was to rotate in the orthopedic and fracture clinics, admit and follow orthopedic patients and would be supervised by Dr. Dennison.

Dr. Spidle, completing his residency in 1968, joined the pathology department at Brackenridge, and practiced there for years.

Dr. Bob Tate had completed his rotating internship at Brackenridge when he was drafted and spent 2 years as a general medical officer at Fort Leonard Wood military base in Missouri. He returned to Brackenridge for a three-year surgical residence with the idea of becoming a general practitioner with a strong surgical component. However, during his third year in 1968, Dr. Maurice Hood called the University of Michigan and arranged for a two-year fellowship in cardiothoracic surgery. After a year in Michigan, Dr. Tate's fourth year of surgery, he was eligible for his general surgery boards. He completed the two-year fellowship and returned to Austin to join the cardiovascular and thoracic group with Dr. Hood. Dr. Tate recalled fondly the teaching skills of Drs. George Tipton, Ben Sims, Dick Lucus, Bob Pape, Maurice Hood, Jim Calhoon, and Hap Arnold while he learned his general surgery techniques at Brackenridge. He appreciated the time spent by Dr. Ferris, a neurosurgeon, who showed him the technique of performing a tracheotomy under local anesthesia in the intensive care unit. He retired from practice in 2000. His hobby over the years involved bird hunting that allowed him the opportunity to hunt in North and South America and in the United Kingdom.

For 1968 the records are not complete as the usual list of residents for the year as generally recorded by the training office. The list of interns is a copy of the National Intern Matching program for Brackenridge; therefore, it does not include the residents. Those interns include Drs. Kenneth O Albers, Bruce M. Bauknight, O. Preston Copland, John A. Craig, Harry A. Croft, Phillip M. Kassner, Daniel M. Kelly, Janusz A. Konikowski, Charles L. Mott, Bert B. Oubre, Benno Anderson, and Oscak Sotelo. Dr. John Craig returned to Galveston, where he had gone to medical school and completed a ophthalmology residency before coming back to Austin to practice. Dr. Charles Mott returned to UTMB for a radiology residency and then settled in Austin.

To complete the 1960's for the training program, the class of 1969 had ten interns and four residents. The interns that year were Drs. Fred Ames, Tarver Bailey, Bill Bass, Charles Hill, Don Howard, Jim McNabb, Fay Mott, Stan Novy, Hayne Sheffield, and Mike Stewart. Dr. McNabb returned to the medical school at Galveston to complete a residency in ophthalmology and nutrition before entering practice back in Austin. The residents that year included Paulo F. L. Becker, second year pathology; Ray Buck, second year surgery; Pierre Greef, second year surgery; and Ken Fannin, who would compete his surgery residency as chief resident. Dr. Fannin joined the surgery practice of Dr. Raleigh Ross and Dr. Tom Coopwood in general surgery. Most of their patients were admitted to Brackenridge.

As the 1970's began, the lists of trainees become longer and I will not include the names of all of the doctors in the program in this part of the text but will put their names in the index for completeness. It is interesting to notice the trend in the class of 1970. There were seven interns and eleven residents. Three of the interns were married and all but one of the residents was married. I note that their living arrangement were all over town, from north to south. There were three who lived in apartments on Lakeshore Drive.

In the 1960's, Brackenridge had the only emergency room in town so, essentially, all of the trauma cases were taken there. That made for very busy general surgery, neurosurgery, and orthopedic services and a great deal of experience for the residents and interns. Obstetrics was handled at the other three hospitals, including St. David's, Seton and Holy Cross but the obstetrical charity care at Brackenridge was busy. Internal medicine had a busy charity and private practice. The pediatric program continued to grow and was supported by almost all of the pediatricians who admitted more and more of their patients to that service.

The 1970's, The Perfect Storm

There was a surprising confluence of conditions and ideas that made the 1970s a very dynamic period in the Austin medical community, particularly at Brackenridge. Those changes would include money, in the form of increasing insurance coverage, including Medicare and Medicaid; internship and residency training program changes; improved emergency medical services, including emergency rooms and ambulance services; increase in the number of medical schools in the state and nation; vastly expanding medical specialization; out-patient surgical centers; and phenomenal population growth. In Austin, a new facility for Brackenridge was built and the old red brick building was destroyed. A new organization was created for the training program. An entirely new emergency room was built in the new Brackenridge building with a full time dedicated staff. The other hospitals in town realized that money could be made from emergency services so they opened new facilities of their own. This required a coordination of the new ambulance service to serve the requirements of those new facilities under consideration. It is interesting to see what happened when the hospital realized that, although ER brought in some charity care, they also brought in paying patients. These multiple new entities created a complex puzzle to be fitted together under the management of politicians, doctors, investment interests, management groups, consultants galore, and the public in general. What a stew pot!

Nationally there were predictions of doctor shortages. In 1965 there were three medical schools in Texas; University of Texas in Galveston, Baylor University College of Medicine in Houston and Southwestern Medical school in Dallas. The legislature got rather busy and created several new medical schools. The University of Texas Medical School in

San Antonio opened in 1966 with its first graduation class in 1970. Most of the students completed their class work in Dallas and Galveston, as the San Antonio facility was not complete. The University of Texas Medical School in Houston opened June 13, 1969. Texas Tech Medical school opened in 1972 and Texas A&M opened in Bryan and Temple in 1977. The Texas College of Osteopathic Medicine was opened in 1970 in Fort Worth. This would greatly increase the number of doctors looking for internship and residency slots in the state of Texas. A number of new medical schools were planned nationally, including a new four-year medical school at the Mayo Clinic opening in 1972.

In an effort to provide for the training of more doctors, the America Medical Association and the Association of America Medical Colleges decided that it would be reasonable to shorten the post graduate training of doctors. Thus they agreed that by 1975 they would not accredit internships that were not integrated into residency training programs. This is the information that Dr. Pape had brought back to the community in 1969. By this method they would attempt to shorten the length of the residency training by a year. A number of different ways were proposed to shorten medical school training but that never caught on at that time. It was under this directive that the program at Brackenridge would be significantly changed over the ensuing years.

It should be noted that on July 30, 1965, Lyndon Johnson signed Medicare and Medicaid into law. This would provide health care coverage for people over sixty-five and for low-income people. This would significantly increase the demand for medical services, exacerbating the predicted shortages of doctors. In 1972, during President Nixon's term, Congress extended Medicare to cover individuals under age sixty-five who had long-term disabilities. As a direct result of the law creating Medicare, payments to hospitals included some portion of that payment for training purposes. Over the years that formula has been modified but this was quite a financial benefit to trainee and teaching staff salaries in hospitals that maintained a training program.

Financing of medical treatment changed dramatically over time. In the 1930's and 1940's doctors struggled to make a living in many practices. Chickens, eggs, and moonshine, which my uncle received in exchange for treatment in central Kentucky in that period, made for rather limited income. More and more businesses were providing health insurance to their employees as a business deductible expense in the

1950's and 1960's. This increased the money going into treatment of patients. Blue Cross and Blue Shield joined forces in 1972 and became a profitable enterprise, although they remained a non-profit organization. Medicare and Medicaid, starting in 1965, pumped large sums of money into the healthcare system in the form of payment for office visits and hospital inpatient care. That increased in 1972 with Medicare payments for patients with disabilities. The growth of treatment options expanded exponentially through the 1970s and 80s resulting in a significant increase in health care costs and inflation. The development of many innovations such as joint replacements, coronary artery bypass and stent surgery, cataract surgery, arthroscopic and laparoscopic surgery, and treatment of premature infants is, in my opinion, a direct result of insurance money pouring into the system and providing support for these many new innovations and surprisingly expensive treatments.

In 1950 the population of Austin was 132,189. It grew 32% in the 1950's, 26% in the 1960's and 27% in the 1970's resulting in a population of 345,890 people in 1980. That meant that there was an increase of 213,600 people as compared to 1950. The demands on Brackenridge hospital were clearly increasing. In the early 1960's, the City Council commissioned a study that ultimately stated that Brackenridge needed to increase to 500 beds and the University of Texas should have a medical school campus across 15th Street. It was recommended that St David's should increase to 250 beds and Seton and Holy Cross should consider combining their facilities. The reader is referred to the book, "Admissions" for a detailed account of the many steps, missteps and slow progress of the building of the new structure of Brackenridge as it stands today. The process would involve several phases and gradual completion of the new hospital.[3]

Of course, those recommendations were not followed particularly closely. Seton moved its location from the University of Texas campus area and constructed a completely new six-story facility on 38th Street, opening in 1975. It certainly did increase the number of beds and improved services. A new dedicated emergency room was part of the hospital with a full time emergency staff. Seton also started a new service referred to as "walk away" surgery or "outpatient surgery". A few years later they acquired Holy Cross Hospital but closed it as its location was not ideal and it was a somewhat odd building, as it was cylindrical.

St. David's Hospital had already moved from Seventeenth Street where it had been managed by St. Davis's Episcopal Church and community doctors since 1924. It's new location, as of 1955, was a five-acre tract on Thirty Second Street. It was partially motivated to move because of the proximity of doctors' offices being built at Medical Arts Square, on the corner of what was then Red River and Nineteenth Street. It had 104 beds, was air conditioned, and had no windows in the operating rooms. This allowed for darkening the rooms and meant less potential contamination from outside air. It was expanded to 268 beds in 1964. In 1978, a large expansion was added on the east side of the main hospital including ancillary services and, shortly after, Park St. David's was constructed to the south with doctor's offices and an outpatient surgical facility, constructed by an outside group of developers. The outpatient surgical center was built, to a certain extent, in response to the opening of Bailey Outpatient Surgical Center in 1973 on the west side of town. It was not until the early 1980's that a dedicated emergency room was added to the main facility on 32nd Street.[27]

There was another concern for which there was much discussion. Brackenridge Nursing School remained an expense for the city. The city fathers discussed discontinuing that program, as there was also a nursing program at the University of Texas. On February 2, 1971, a resolution by the Travis County Medical Society was passed, encouraging the City to continue support of the nursing school. Most of the doctors that used Brackenridge felt that the quality of nursing by those student graduates was excellent, and certainly competitive with the University of Texas students. The School of Nursing administration was financially part of the budget of Brackenridge hospital. There were dorm rooms and a cafeteria to support. In 1974, the administrator, Mr. Brown, recommended that the management of the nursing school be transferred to the newly opened Austin Community College (ACC). This would save $500,000 from the hospital budget. The hospital board and then the City Council approved the transfer, so that in September of 1974 the Brackenridge School of Nursing was transferred to ACC. The third or clinical year of training would continue to be at Brackenridge, as well as some time to be spent at St. David's Hospital.

The City of Austin began a new direction of growth for Brackenridge. A building plan was developed and bond elections were held in 1964.

This would begin a slow, painful, protracted course of design, building, controversy, missteps and problems, the flames of which would be fanned by the news media who expressed little understanding of the process and whose only interest seemed to be conflict. The project was bound to be expensive compared to the history of slow additions to the building and staff that had occurred over the past 50 years. The major issue that provided the greatest angst was the decision about who in the community was responsible for care of the poor. In most major communities across the country, the county has been primarily responsible for charity care. Austin was unique in that it had been running the city hospital for the past seventy years. There was little question in the medical community as to who would do the hands on care. The doctors in Austin had been taking care of the indigent patients and they planned to continue that responsibility. The major expense would fall to the City of Austin. There was even discussion in the political community and among movers and shakers in the 1970's that the City of Austin might sell or lease the hospital to an independent entity who could manage the hospital, include charity care, and also make a profit. There were some interesting meetings at Brackenridge regarding discussion of some of these possibilities. Some of us thought that making Brackenridge profitable would be like selling the Salvation Army or Goodwill to someone who would make it a profitable. It was hard to take these plans seriously. All of those possibilities drifted away in the heat of the night and the City plodded through in a somewhat less than a streamlined fashion, but, indeed, got the job done.

The overall plan was to build the new hospital immediately west of the old red brick facility that had been in use for seventy years. Construction was to be completed in phases, as money was always an issue. Starting in 1967 with phase 1A, a hole in the ground was dug for a large base to the building and a tower with floors four, five, and six completed and the seventh shelled in, as the first step. The seventh floor would be completely finished out later. There was a need for beds in the first phase and that is where things started. That section was completed in October, 1970. Again the news media fanned the flames of dissent, charging that if new beds were opened in the new tower and beds were closed in the old brick building, the poor would not have adequate beds. That was, of course, complete nonsense as there never was any interruption of services to any patient.

There was a significant push by the medical community at Brackenridge and the Travis County Medical Society to keep pushing the plan for completion. In an effort to provide some logic to the debate, Dr. Bud Dryden ran for and was elected to the City Council with the stated objective to support the completion of the new hospital. He was also supportive of the Brackenridge School of Nursing that was financed by the city.

To add fuel to the multiple controversies, Mr. Ben Tobias resigned as the administrator and was replace by Mr. William K. Brown. Mr. Brown's smooth, Marine Corps manner is illustrated in his dealing with Dr. Georgia Legett and her clinic patients, noted earlier in this text. He had limited people skills but was a skilled administrator. With all this controversy surrounding the hospital there was a significant test to the energy, loyalty and compassion of the medical community. Some of the staff moved their loyalty to other hospitals in the area for various reasons. The newly completed Seton and St. David's facilities that were convenient to office locations, the changing dynamics of specialty care, and the requirement that doctors provide emergency room coverage when on staff influenced many decisions.

As if there weren't enough problems, politics was a significant problem. During this process of planning and building from 1964 to completion in 1978 there were six different mayors including Lester Palmer, Harry Akins, Travis LaRue, Roy Butler, Jeffrey Friedman, and Carole Keeton McClellen; a number of changes on the city council; and three city managers, Lynn H. Andrews, R. A. Tinstman, and Dan Davidson. There were frightful discussions of maintaining the hospital, who would be blamed if bonds were proposed to the citizens, and what would be the political fall out. There were the advocates for the poor and minorities and a desire to keep private inpatients to offset losses. All of this was under the dubious scrutiny of the news media that kept the politicians worried and confused their logic.

In 1972 money was added to the coffers for construction and in 1974 phase 2A was started. This included finishing out the shelled-in 7th floors of the tower, constructing the lower floors to contain the laboratory, physical therapy and other ancillary services plus adding the shells of floors eight and nine. That was completed in 1976, bringing the bed count to 344. From 1976 through 1978, Brackenridge experienced a significant reduction in income and occupancy. It is likely that much of that had to do with all the controversy, the new Seton hospital being completed, and the number of doctors choosing to switch admissions to Seton and St. David's. Mr. William Brown left as administrator in 1977 and Mr. Bob Spurk, the assistant administrator, became acting administrator. Mr. Spurk had started his residency in management at Brackenridge in 1972 and was then hired as assistant administrator. In 1977 he became acting administrator and then full administrator in 1978. Much to the credit of Bob Spurk, who worked with the community, talked to civic groups, and courted the doctors in 1978, the occupancy rate was up to 90%, income was much improved, and phase 2B was completed. Phase 2B included the completion of the emergency room, laboratory facilities, the new surgical area and the intensive care unit. Floors eight and nine were also completed. Most of the services were now in the new building. Money was secured to complete the structure, and the old red brick building was demolished. The new hospital now had many of the needed beds on bright, cheery floors with wide halls, wonderful large operating rooms, a highly efficient emergency room, new space for ancillary services of x-ray and laboratory, and a uniquely cheerful administrator in Bob Spurk. A major problem for him was the necessity to spend hours at the city council meetings and away from the hospital, so that he would be available to speak to the council when his turn came to discuss needs of the hospital. There was no provision for timing his appearances and he waited at the pleasure of the council to make his presentations. In 1984 he left Brackenridge to work for the Austin Diagnostic Clinic. The new administrator was Mr. John Dandridge. Mr. Tom Young followed him and was a very effective administrator. Running the hospital was difficult, dealing with the city bureaucracy, balancing the budget with charity costs with paying patients, and dealing with the ever-demanding needs for medical care and new equipment.[28]

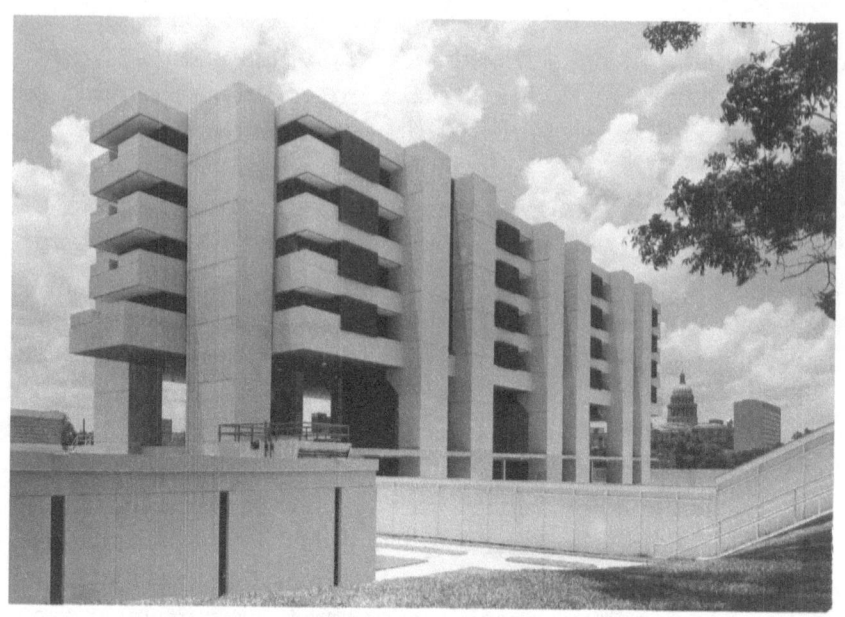

Early work on completing the seven-story tower (with permission, Austin History Center, Austin Public Library.)

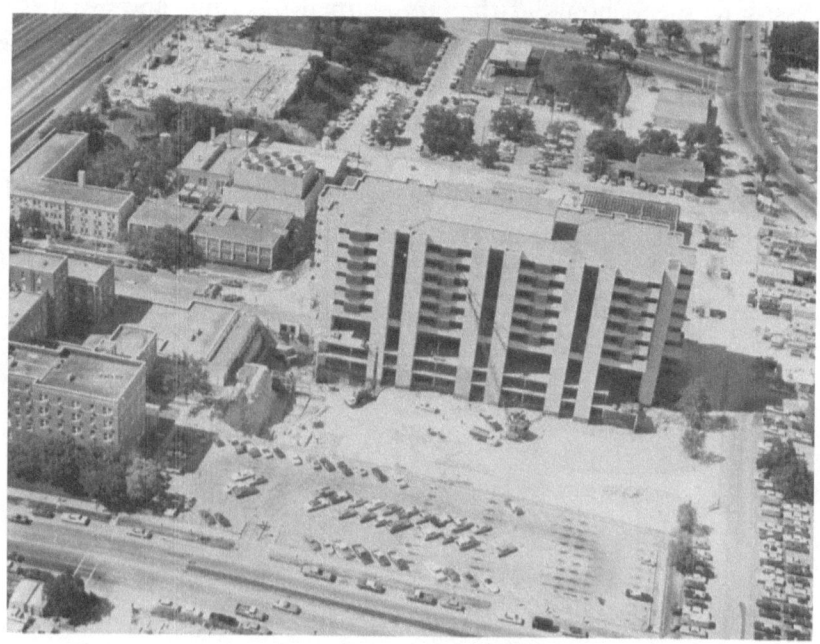

Progress on finishing out floor 8 and 9 (with permission, Austin History Center, Austin Public Library.)

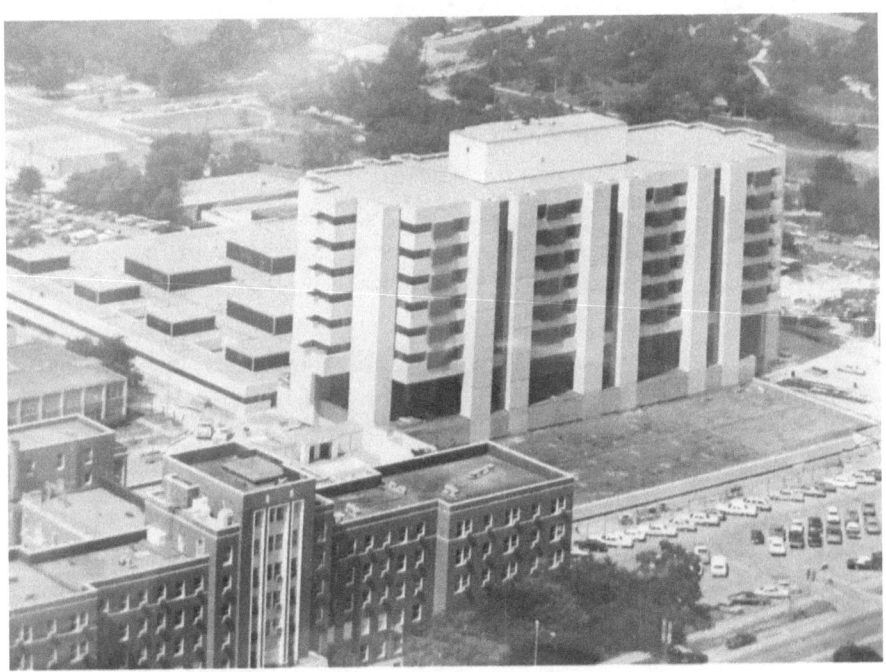

Completed emergency room, ICU and laboratories in the first floor and basement to south of tower and ancillary services to the north. (with permission, Austin History Center, Austin Public Library.)

Central Texas Medical Foundation

The earliest suggestion that a foundation be considered under the umbrella of the Travis County Medical Society was at the June 8th, 1971 meeting of the society. Dr. Robert Exline proposed that a Travis County Foundation for Medical Care be established, similar to one in Denver, Colorado. It's purpose would be to negotiate contracts with private insurance companies and the federal government (on behalf of local doctors). This was partially in response to issues with insurance companies and meaningful standards for health plans. It was later in that year that the federal government established the first price/wage freeze for Medicare under the Nixon Administration. As the ideas evolved for the formation of a foundation, it was proposed by Dr. Fred Vogt, in January, 1972, that improvements in emergency medical care be considered as one of the goals. Dr. Bob Dennison became the chairman of the emergency room committee at Brackenridge and he would be very involved in improving the ER at Brackenridge. It was recorded in the TCMS minutes that there was to be a symposium in Houston on emergency medical care sponsored by the American College of Surgeons and the American College of Emergency Physicians. This was to coincide with the proposal that federal funds for the development of emergency medical services and ambulance services might be available.

It was also proposed by Dr. Thomas Kirksey that medical education, involving the internship and residency program, be included in the goals for a foundation. Dr. Kirksey was the chairman of the medical education program committee at Brackenridge in 1972. He had come to Austin in 1969 to join Dr. Hood, Arnold, and Calhoon in their cardiothoracic and vascular practice. He spent many hours working on the transition from the old medical education system and encouraging the organization of the future Central Texas Medical Foundation. As the chairman of the Education Committee at Brackenridge he actually became the director of medical education as Dr. Pape made a transition to the emergency services. Along with Dr. Hood, Dr. Tom Kirksey was instrumental in developing the emergency medical service and providing training to the new emergency medical technicians. Dr. Daryl Faubion was the Travis County Medical Society president that year and presided over these discussions and organizational developments.

On March 28th, 1972, at a special called meeting of the Board of Directors of the Travis County Medical Society, Dr. Homer (Hap) Arnold made a motion, seconded by Dr. Grover Bynum, "that the articles of incorporation for the Central Texas Medical Foundation, or whatever name is acceptable by the Secretary of State, and the Board of Director be accepted," and that the articles be referred to Mr. Overton, TMA legal council, for processing and incorporation. Officers for the foundation were to be Lobdell Exline, M.D., president; Thomas Kirksey, M.D., vice president; Ernest C. Butler, M.D., secretary; Alford Hazzard, M.D. treasurer; and Terry Collier, M. D. assistant secretary-treasurer. Other members of the board included Grover L. Bynum; M. D., Ted L. Edwards, M.D.; Lansing Thorne, M.D.; and Hardy Thompson, M.D., immediate past president of the medical society. Mr. John Kemp was the executive director of the medical society at the time.[29]

The articles of incorporation of The Central Texas Medical Foundation were recorded on May 3, 1972. A summary of the Articles is included and the complete document is provided in the appendix of this book. The purposes as stated in the articles included: "(a) To promote, develop, define and encourage medical education and the distribution of medical health services and care by its members to the people of Travis County and the Central Texas area. (b) To supervise, manage and administer for its members any health plans or similar arrangements; (c) To foster, encourage and coordinate the establishment of uniform standards of medical care and health services amongst other similar foundations; (d) to Provide members and the general public standards for reviewing disputes or grievances; (e) To keep records relative to medical services; (f) To negotiate contracts; (g) To purchase, acquire or lease real property; (h) To apply for or purchase rights or privileges from government agencies; (i) To carry out activities deemed proper to promote the interests of the foundation members; (j) To carry out any part of the foregoing objects and purposes to attain or further any of its objects or purposes." This document was signed by Dr. Darrell Faubion, Dr. Hardy Thompson, and Dr. Grover Bynum.

In this manner the first and only organization in the country was formed by a medical society for the express purpose of organizing a new medical training system, establishing a new ambulance service, managing contracts with health care payers, and managing the staff of an improved full time emergency room. The Travis County Medical Society was unique in taking on the responsibility of training but, in doing so, would, with the aid of private practice physicians in the community, contribute to the quality of care to the indigent patients and of patients who had not established a relationship with a doctor in town. The latter group was classified as non-preference cases.

To obtain further information on how the medical education might be organized, Dr. Kirksey and Dr. Pape made a trip to Pensacola, Florida to observe a program there organized for training. There they found a great deal of support by community doctors for a program in which several hospitals would come together to organize the local training program. Their plan seemed to have achieved accreditation and was progressing in the direction that Austin needed to go. They returned home to encourage progress by the Central Texas Medical Foundation.[30]

With the organization of the Central Texas Medical Foundations (CTMF) there was now a mechanism by which progress could be made in several directions. On the top of the list was the development of the training program. In addition there was the need to organize the emergency room, especially as the interns were going to be less available for patient care. This would be a three-pronged approach with the development of full time doctors to cover the treatment in the ER, reorganization of the intern and resident coverage in the ER, and development of the ambulance service or emergency medical service to serve the peripheral emergency needs. As mentioned earlier, there was a national meeting in Houston with the primary goal of improving ambulance or emergency medical services. This meeting would emphasize guidelines for emergency medical services in general.

Ambulance Service

It was during those early years, 1971 to 1972 that another committee was established by the Travis County Medical Society to discuss the ambulance services in Austin. The only services available then were provided by the funeral homes and the Austin Ambulance service, a private contractor. The committee included chairman Curtis Weeks, civil service director for the City; Morris Hohman and Joe Manor, both funeral home directors; Dr. Pape and members of the medial society. It is noted that the City had made a contract with Mr. Dale Owens, owner of the Austin Ambulance Service in the late 1960's. As a member of the committee, Bob Pape accompanied the head of the City transportation department to Dallas and to Tulsa, Oklahoma to study their EMS services. He, along with city council members, Dr. Bud Dryden and Burle Handcock, went to Jacksonville, Florida to look at their operations and equipment.

As a City, and possibly a County-run process, there were many committees. Mr. Mike Levy, Editor of the Texas Monthly Magazine, and a self appointed expert on quality of City services and efficiencies, was selected to head a Quality Assurance Committee to evaluate the various possibilities. He was very interested in elements of the Dallas system as a model for Austin. Interestingly, all of the "systems" in place were quite new, as these emergency systems had been in place for only a few years. When Bob Pape went to the Washington, D. C. American College of Emergency Physicians (ACEP) meeting, he visited with Arlington, Virginia personnel who demonstrated makes and models of ambulances as well as radio systems that had only been in use about a year. All ambulances were modified hearse vehicles at the time and the manufacturers were developing new models to respond to the national interest in emergency services.

Bob Pape also attended the State ACEP organizational meeting in Dallas at The Texas Medical Association annual meeting in 1973. In October, 1974, Travis County Medical Society officers Bob Exline, Tom Kirksey, V. C. Smart, and Bob Dennison were instrumental in sending Bob to that national ACEP meeting in Washington D.C. Interestingly, during that meeting, Bob stayed in a small hotel room under a standing reservation of Fred Vogt. Mr. Vogt was a Nixon appointee from Boerne, Texas to a select White House committee on EMS. During that visit to Washington, Bob was asked to make contact with Dr. R. R. Hannas in order to offer a visit/interview for a possible appointment to a position as director of the ER in Austin. Dr. R. R. Hannas was the immediate past president of the America College of Emergency Physicians.[26]

Developing the emergency room and ambulance service would require jumping some interesting hurdles. One would expect that losing ambulance business to a new service would meet with some resistance from the funeral directors, as that had been some source of income. I certainly recall some discussion of that issue at the time, but it became apparent that the requirement for an emergency medical service was going to be well beyond the capabilities of the funeral directors and, therefore, this issue did not continue as a major problem.

The Fire Department is owned and managed by the city, the traditional management relationship in most communities. Their services are available primarily within the city limits. Emergency medical services tend to involve a much larger geographic area. Brackenridge primarily, but other Austin hospitals as well, had provided care for patients from all over central Texas, including locations near Columbus to the east, Burnet to the north, Dripping Springs and Wimberley to the west and beyond San Marcos to the south. Hospital facilities in Austin were much larger and provided more advanced care than could be possible in the smaller surrounding communities. Thus ambulances brought patients from many surrounding cities for care.

At issue was whether the service would be part of the Austin Fire Department or whether it would be a separate entity. This issue was perhaps only slightly less important than whether we would have the money and interest to create a new emergency service at all. Nationally, there were a number of ambulance services integrated into the fire departments. The firemen were trained in first aid and rescue and already had a lot of equipment for rescue around the city. They expected to be called to fire emergencies but also to automobile accidents and other sites where injuries were encountered. There was a debate nationally as to which direction communities should follow to provide the best of care and services. What if the fire department was involved in a major fire and then was required to respond to a heart attack or motor vehicle accident elsewhere? And, in Austin, one of the major proponents in the medical community that was lobbying for an improved emergency service was Dr. Maurice Hood. As noted earlier, he was the son of a fireman, retained a lifelong interest in the fire department, had an emergency radio in his home and auto, and responded to fires on frequent occasions. He was very supportive of the position that the emergency medical services should be part of the Fire Department. He had actually been involved in the early training of Austin firefighters in first aid, resuscitation, and rescue.

To put this development into some historical perspective, it should be noted that it was not until 1971 that the Houston Fire Department took over the ambulance service after years of ambulances being provided by funeral homes, Jefferson Davis Hospital and some volunteer organizations. In the 1960's the Grady Memorial Hospital in Atlanta, Georgia ran the ambulance service staffed by medical students who had some first aid training. The City of Memphis commissioned the Fire Department to establish a city-wide ambulance service in 1965. In 1968 the Fort Worth Ambulance service was privately owned under contract with the City and the attendants completed a three-day course provided by the American Academy of Orthopedic Surgeons, as well as American Red Cross Standard and Advanced First Aid course. The service remained a private company until the late 1970, when the City took over. Fort Worth followed very closely the development of services in Dallas. Austin was clearly in the middle of the changes that were occurring in the state and the nation. National emergency medical service standards had been established in the late 1960s.[30]

An independent emergency service would require its own bureaucracy, management team, and physical locations for equipment and personnel. This would involve building separate buildings to house the ambulances, but, of course, garages near the fire department would be needed if that department managed the ambulances. An independent

EMS would require the assistance of the fire department when certain equipment was needed, such as the "jaws of life," a device invented in the 1960's.

Historically the actual ambulance vehicle was evolving. In the 1950s and 1960 the vehicle most commonly seen was a modified Cadillac automobile converted to the shape of a station wagon with doors on the back to allow loading a stretcher or a coffin. Chevrolet station wagons were also modified. In the late 1960s, Chevrolet Suburban trucks were modified, with the addition of lights and sirens for the purpose. It was not until 1970 that the "Modular" ambulance/truck was produced with headroom, side compartments for equipment and a full lighting system that would meet new federal standards for ambulance construction. In the budget records of the early Austin EMS, the cost of the first ambulance was $21,329. So, the creation of an emergency ambulance service required management, trained personnel, specialized equipment, a dispatch headquarters, radios for communication, and many things that were evolving in our community and across the country.[31]

Ultimately the City of Austin elected to be responsible for this new service and created a service separate from the Fire Department. On January 1, 1976 Austin EMS was established as a non-civil service municipal department. There were initially 32 employees and the ambulances were operated with personnel equipped with Basic Life Support training. Drs. Hood, Dr. Kirksey and many others were involved in training personnel. Apparently, some of the training was done by emergency room nurses who also had basic life support training. Dr. Pape, in addition to his work in the emergency room, was on the committee to set up the new Emergency Medical Service. He was the medical director for three years and was involved in training several classes of paramedics. Drs. Kirksey, Hood, Pape and others set up continuing education classes, interviewed new applicants and did periodic "stress testing" of the crews to make sure they maintained their proficiency. Dr. Pape and others trained about 300 emergency medical technicians (EMTs) during his tenure. He rode in some ambulances on his days off from the emergency room to get acquainted with the new process. New buildings in the community were to be built to house the employees and the equipment for the new ambulance service. These were located all over town and ultimately some were housed in fire stations. The first separate headquarters facility was on Red River

Street, just south of Brackenridge Hospital. The building now houses the Brick Oven Restaurant.[26,31]

In 1980 the personnel riding in the ambulances were further trained to a tiered system where some were Advanced Life Support trained (ALS) while the rest were Basic Life Support (BLS) trained. In 1996 the system involved having all personnel trained at the ALS level and were called paramedics; however in 2012 the system was returned to the tiered system as it was just not possible to continue to recruit enough paramedics trained at the ALS level.

The list of early medical directors for the program included Drs. Bob Pape, Bob Anderson (cardiology), Don Patrick (neurosurgery), and Pat Crocker (emergency Medicine). The first full time medical director was Dr. Racht in 1995. Early managing directors were William Lever, Bill Bullock, and Sue Edwards.[26]

It was not until 1985 that the helicopter service called "Star Flight" was added to the emergency medical services in Austin. This project was a joint project of Brackenridge Hospital, which supplied the nurses, the City, the EMS, which provided the medics, and the County, which supplied the pilots. That service has moved beyond simple transportation of the injured or acutely ill. Star Flight is involved in some fire fighting, rescue operations on land and water, and wilderness search and rescue. In 2009 Star Flight separated from the Austin EMS and became a department of Travis County.[31]

Improving the Emergency Room

Creation of a new emergency room would require completion of the hospital started in 1967. The emergency room in 1972 remained in the annex on the south side of the old red brick building. It was really the hall that connected the old red brick hospital building to the new building. The completion of the ground floor in the Brackenridge hospital tower, including the emergency room, would have to wait until 1977. The management of the emergency room staff of doctors by the Central Texas Medical Foundation would be a unique arrangement in the United States. All other cities managed their staff through the hospital itself or the training program under the guidance of a medical school. Bob Pape was made coordinator between the medical education office, where he was the director, and the organization of the emergency room doctors, where staffing was primarily the interns. That was July 1, 1971. At the July 17, 1972 meeting of the CTMF, Dr. Exline announced that Dr. Dennison had volunteered to be the chairman of the emergency room committee and to arrange seminars on emergency services. He was also planning to develop standard operating procedure manuals for the ER.[26]

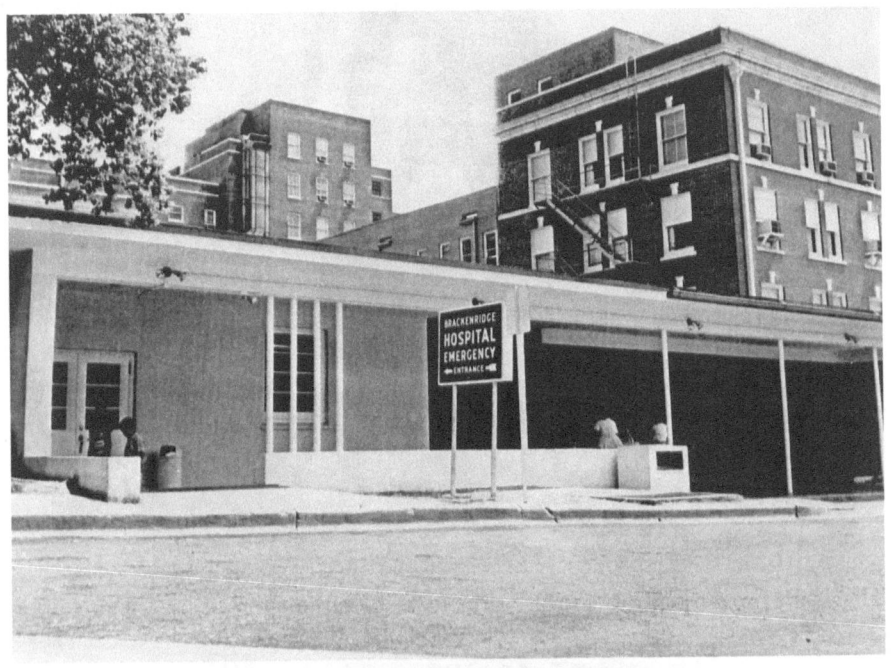

Emergency room and clinic area on south side
of the old red brick Brackenridge.

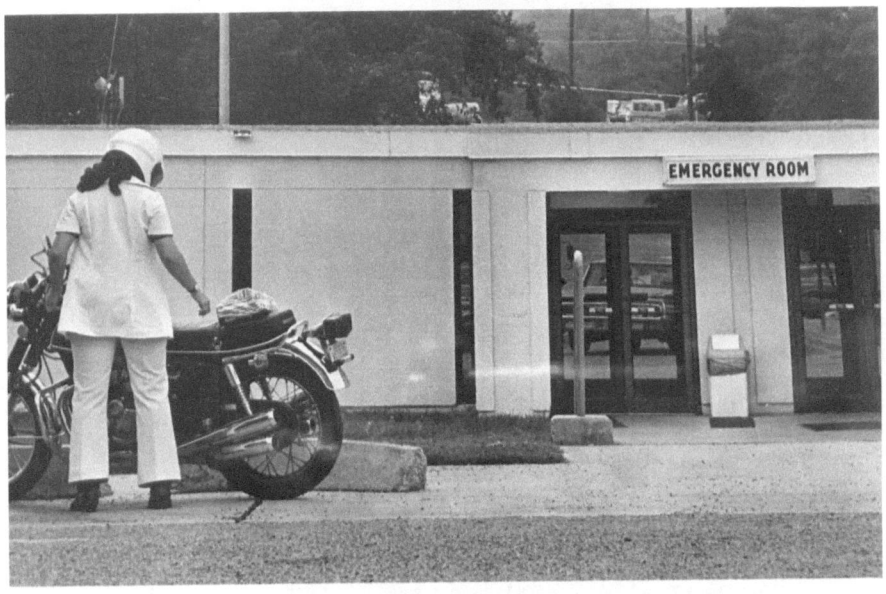

Emergency room entrance.

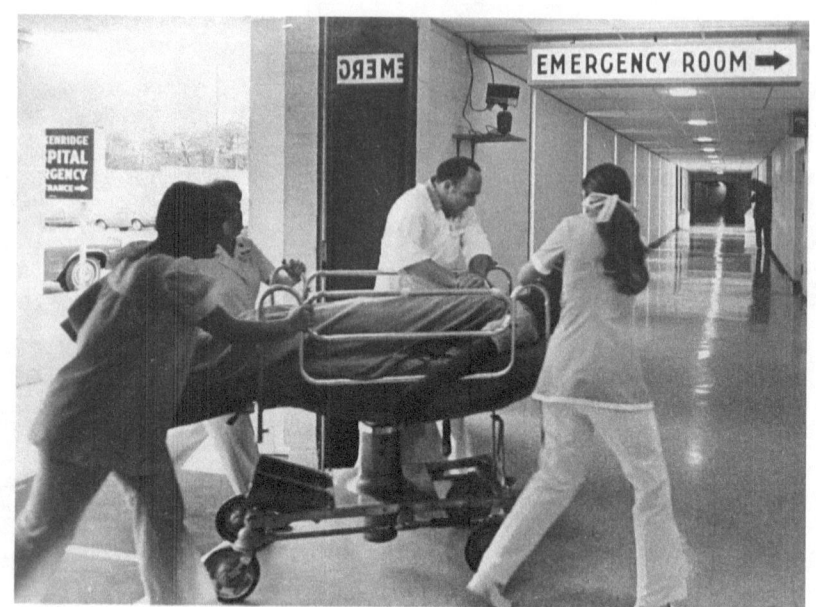
Patient on a stretcher being brought into the hall of the emergency room.

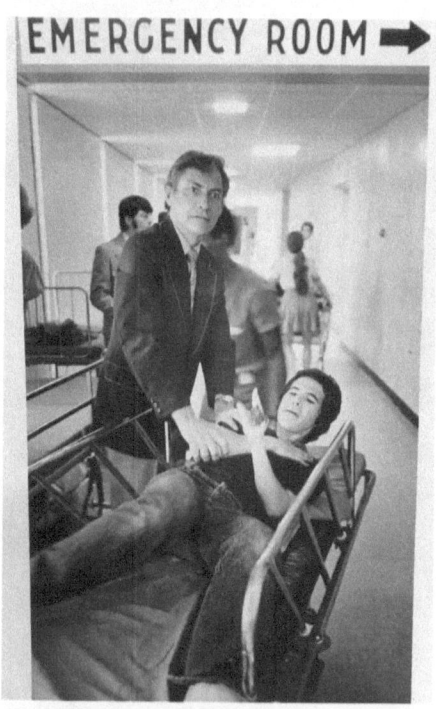
Dr. Roy Leaman providing triage in a drill for mock mass disaster in emergency room with simulated patient.

Most of the interns were removed from ER rotations in 1973 to comply with the American Medical Association's rulings on internship rotations. There was a six-month period when there was very limited house staff coverage for the ER. Sometimes there were large gaps between some intern rotations. The interns, residents, the city physician, and community doctors had covered the ER for the last 40 years. Doctor members of the new Central Texas Medial Foundation volunteered to take shifts in the ER. Dr. Pape was asked to schedule some doctors for coverage and was assigned the task of coordinating between the training program, the house staff and the emergency room. It was a somewhat disappointing and slow process to find adequately trained and willing staff for the ER. It was quite challenging for the medical society to provide coverage, as the members all had active practices to maintain. A sign up schedule was established by which the doctors would be assigned a shift to be covered. It was set up so that there were generally two doctors per shift. Dr. Pape noted that a number of the assigned doctors did not show up for their shifts. He also noted that some doctors had little experience in the ER and he personally needed to back them up. Covering an office practice in medicine, pediatrics or obstetrics, or even ophthalmology, urology or orthopedic surgery, was quite different from covering a general emergency room with acute pediatric, medicine, surgery, or psychiatric emergencies.[26]

I came to Austin in the summer of 1971. My training had included a rotating internship, including the standard medicine, surgery, obstetrics and pediatric rotations. I had a year of general surgery before my orthopedics and had also spent two years in the Public Health Service on an Indian Reservation. That experience in the Indian Health Service involved a very busy general medicine practice, also including pediatrics and delivery of about 60 babies over the two years. I was also a new member of the CTMF in 1973 when the ER problems became apparent. I covered some rotations in the ER and found that most of the problems were pretty routine, but I had very little experience with psychological problems and medication. I depended on the nursing staff for some significant back up, including keeping me informed about what the indications were for some medications.

One of the nurses on whom I depended was Mrs. Leida Bryce. She was a graduate of the Brackenridge School of Nursing and had been the nurse supervisor in the emergency room for twenty-seven years.

With an emergency room volume of about 41,000 visits per year and an outpatient clinic volume of 26,000, it was a busy place. Considering that the ER and the clinics were housed in the same hallway structure on the south side of the main hospital building, it is remarkable that it functioned at all. It was certainly crowded.

Dr. Don Patrick, a neurosurgeon, and Dr. Charlie Felger, an internist with subspecialty in gastroenterology, covered some rotations together. Dr. Felger told me that he saw the medical problems and Dr. Patrick saw the surgical patients. He said that after seeing some patient he and Don would say to the patients, "the fee for the ER visit was $15." Many of the patients would have no money or would say they only had $3 or $5. Dr. Felger would say, "that will cover the visit." He might go home with $15 in his pocket and call it a successful night. Most of the rest of us did not have the fortitude to request a fee and would assign any monies to the TCMF.[33]

Dr. John Boyd completed his internship at Brackenridge in 1973 and had rotated through the ER. He went to medical school in Galveston and had come to Austin to do an externship with Dr. Moncreif in nephrology. He also did rotations in urology and with Dr. Felger in internal medicine. This experience led him to his internship in Austin. Following his internship he had made arrangements to join the practice of Dr. John Kelly and Dr. Joe Reneau in general practice. They did not have room, physically, for him in their office at the time. As a consequence, he signed on to work in the emergency room for six to twelve months. Early in his work, a patient was brought to the ER with a scalp laceration. On further evaluation, he was noted to have a very rapid pulse and low blood pressure. He also had no breath sounds on one side of the chest. A chest x-ray confirmed a hemo-pneumothorax. Dr. Boyd put in a chest tube and got back a large amount of blood. With an extremely ill patient and no blood immediately available, he and Dr. Howard Hachman auto transfused the patient with blood from his chest tube. The patient benefited from the blood and was take to the intensive care unit, where he did well. Dr. Hachman was working in the ER waiting for a residency position in internal medicine in San Antonio. For a year, Drs. Boyd and Hachman were two of the first full time ER doctors at Brackenridge.[34] Hiring these doctors relieved the problem of doctors covering the ER so that the community doctors were relieved from some of those duties without regular interns covering. I, personally, was quite happy to see that responsibility terminated.

In 1973, Dr. Ben Sims, a general surgeon on the staff, took over management of the emergency room at the request of the emergency room committee. Dr. Sims got quite a surprise one day working in the ER. There were always lots of good stories coming out of that service. On this occasion a woman presented with abdominal pain. The routine, in addition to the history and abdominal exam, would be to do a pelvic exam since pelvic inflammatory disease (PID, usually a sexually transmitted disease) was a common cause of abdominal pain. He requested that the nurse set the patient up on an examining room table for the pelvic exam. Much to his surprise, the "she" was a "he" transvestite and came with the wrong anatomy for a pelvic exam. Ben Sims eventually left that position because of the many difficulties working with the City relative to management and financing the emergency room.

It was not easy to find trained emergency room doctors. There were only two or three residency programs for emergency medicine doctors in the country at the time. The ACEP was providing emergency medicine specialty certification, under a grandfathering process, to physicians who had experience working in an emergency room and also had specialty training in an area that would normally function in an emergency room, such as surgery, internal medicine, and pediatrics. Emergency medicine was not an accepted specialty by the American Board of Medical Specialties at the time.

In the summer of 1973, Dr. Norman Chenven completed his two-year stint in the U. S. Public Health service on a Navajo Indian reservation in Tuba City, Arizona. His experience there in general medicine was very busy in association with 16-18 other doctors in various specialties. He did not have a solid plan for the next step. He had completed medical school in Brooklyn, New York and then an internship in San Antonio. Norm's wife wanted to work on a PhD in history and felt that the University of Texas in Austin would be a good choice. She was accepted to the program so Norm called the student health service at the University of Texas to see if they had a position. They had just filled a position, but the doctor there suggested that he call Dr. Dennison, chairman of the emergency room committee, who was looking for doctors to work. He talked to Dr. Dennison by phone and set up an interview. The night before the interview Norm had a unique experience. On the reservation the Indian males routinely wore their hair in a ponytails and Norm had adopted that style. He insisted that he was not from a hippy background. Norm's wife said that in her view the ponytail would not be considered favorably for the interview in the morning. She got the scissors out, cut his ponytail off, and tried to smooth up the haircut. He had the interview the next day and was hired. Some time later, Dr. Dennison admitted to Norm that he had wondered about his haircut, as it seemed rather rough at the time.[35]

In 1974, Dr. Chenven was asked to be interim director as Dr. Pape was becoming quite busy with the training program and also dealing with the development of the emergency medical service. Dr. Chenven served in that position until Dr. R. R. Hannas was hired to be director. During that period Drs. Bill Bass, Tom Daniels, Dick Berry, and Sidney Robins joined the staff as full time emergency doctors.

Between 1975 and 1976 Dr. R. R. Hannas, who had been interviewed in Washington, D.C. by Dr. Pape, became the director of the ER and he was there when Dr. Don Connell was hired to work full time. Dr. Connell was a 1970 University of Texas at Austin graduate who completed medical school at the University of Texas, Southwestern in 1974. He completed a year of surgery at Baylor Hospital in Dallas and then came to Austin to do graduate studies in neurophysiology. To support himself he signed up for a one half time schedule in the emergency room while doing the graduate work. In 1976 he dropped the graduate work, as it was just too much to keep up with, and he became full time in the ER. He worked with Drs. Tom Daniels, Sidney Robins (Brackenridge trained), Richard Berry, Norm Chenven and Bob Pape.

Dr. Connell worked in the Brackenridge ER for almost ten years until he, along with Dr. Blewett and Dr. Brooks Boch formed a group to cover the emergency room at St. David's. He related an incident that bolstered his confidence working in the emergency room. A patient came in with a head injury and changes in blood pressure such that he was concerned about a intra-abdominal injury as well as the head injury. Dr. Donald Patrick was the neurosurgeon on call and came in to see the patient. Dr. Patrick promptly took the patient to surgery for his head injury. Dr. Connell was pretty sure he himself had not made the correct decision relative to care of the patient. After the surgery was completed, Dr. Patrick returned to the emergency room and, in a very kind and patient way, explained what to look for in a patient with multiple trauma, including a head injury. Dr. Patrick had evaluated many such patients in an evacuation hospital in Viet Nam, so had extensive experience with this type of patient. Don was so thoroughly impressed by Dr. Patrick's teaching and patience that it bolstered his feelings about continuing in the field of emergency medicine.[36]

At that time each of the services, including medicine, surgery, pediatrics, etc. had a rotating call schedule that provided community doctors as consultants. They also admitted patients who required inpatient care for whatever reason. These patients, referred to a "non-preference patients," usually did not have a personal doctor whom they had seen in the past. This provided back up care to the emergency room doctors and admission for continued care of patients that needed hospitalization. Those services that had residents and teaching responsibilities admitted most of the patients, but care requiring expertise in urology, ophthalmology, orthopedics, plastic surgery and ear, nose, and throat surgery were covered by community doctors. These private doctors admitted patients to themselves and cared for those patients. As these services did not have residents or interns assigned, they would eventually follow the patients in their offices after discharge if necessary. Some would be followed in the Brackenridge clinic system or in city medicine clinics if they had no insurance. All of the services had a specialty clinic arrangement at Brackenridge where patients would be seen for follow up. The specialty clinics were covered by community doctors who took turns, generally a month or two at a time, running those weekly clinics.

The organization of the ER became more complicated in the later 1970s. For that period from 1973 to 1977 Brackenridge had Dr. Pape, Dr. Sims, Dr. Hannas, and the Emergency Room Committee, under CTMF, supervising the emergency room. Dr. Hannas was hired because it was felt that, as a national figure, he might have more clout with the City Council regarding budget discussions. Dr. Hannas was eventually asked to leave the director position when some doctors believed "that he was an untrustworthy politician who was engineering a "take over" of the whole city emergency system."[35]

Dr. Sims returned to the job for a short time to help with the management. In 1976 Drs. Norm Chenven, Tom Daniels, Sidney Robins, and Richard Berry left the emergency room to start a practice together. They set up an office in the Bailey Surgical Center building that housed the first stand-alone outpatient surgical center in Austin. Norm felt that they developed a very nice practice together. However, he had liked the multispecialty model that was present in the Indian Health Service. After some deliberation and study, he left that practice in 1980 to start a multispecialty practice that became the Austin Regional Clinic. Over the ensuing thirty-five years, his clinic would grow to include twenty-one locations over Austin and Round Rock.[35]

The loss of Dr. Chenven and colleagues left as the core group Drs. Ken Sherman (Brackenridge internship), Al Lindsey, Bob Raley, Carl Pevoto, and Don Connell. They were later joined by Dr. Brooks Bock on the team. They worked closely together, had a good esprit de corps, improved patient services, and provided very good coverage for the department.

In that group, Al Lindsey arrived in 1977 just after the new ER opened. He graduated from Southwestern Medical School in Dallas, followed by a year if internal medicine internship in Seattle, 21 months in the Army Medical crops (18 months in Saigon), and then an emergency medicine residency in Dallas at Parkland and the Dallas Veterans Administration hospital. He then did 4 years of emergency medicine in Santa Rosa, California, and then Kaiser Hospital in Marin County. In 1977 he came to Austin and spent two years at Brackenridge before finally settling into a Family Medicine practice in Austin for thirty-four years.[37]

On April 1, 1977 the new emergency room was completed and the service was moved from the hall in the old hospital, where they had ten rooms, to the new Brackenridge Tower that had fourteen rooms. The rooms were larger, much lighter, and there was a much better registration area, social service office, and other ancillary facilities that made the working conditions superb compared to the old area.

For financial, organizational and personnel reasons it seemed logical to consider having an outside organization run that service. They could take on the responsibility for hiring their own physicians and manage the care under close supervision. This was to follow a national trend in emergency room management. There was a significant increase in trained emergency medicine doctors available to contract and provide coverage across the country. It was increasingly complex for private doctors on a committee of the CTMF to manage the changes necessary in the ER. CTMF started looking at various possible companies. From the early 1970's, when few trained emergency medicine doctors were available, to the late 70's when there were some rather large groups available to cover emergency room care, even on a national level, there was an incredible change in medical practice.

There were several groups available to Austin for this function and some ruminating about whom would get the contract. Included in those companies that seemed interested in the Austin contract were Em-Care, Fischer-Mangold, and a couple of others.

Dr. John Blewett moved from Pennsylvania to Austin in September of 1977 because the weather was just "too cold up north." He had competed medical school in Albany in 1971, finished a surgical residency, and was inducted into the Air Force from 1975 to 1977. While in the Air Force he moonlighted in an emergency room under the management of a group called Fisher-Mangold. After moving to Austin and working in the emergency room, he was contacted by Fischer-Mangold to see if he could make the presentation to Central Texas Medical Foundation regarding a potential contract to manage the ER. Since he had worked for their organization while in the military and was now in Austin, it seemed a natural request. They also offered him the opportunity to be the director of the local ER group coverage, if they got the contract. During the negotiations and contract discussions, Dr. Homer Goehrs, the then president of the Travis Medical Society, called Dr. Blewett and confronted him about his association with Fisher-Mangold. Dr. Goehrs was concerned that there was a conflict of interest in promoting Fisher-Mangold while Dr. Goehr thought Dr. Blewett was an employee of CTMF. Dr. Goehrs suggested that Dr. Blewett should leave town. (An old Texas tradition) Dr. Blewett retorted that he was, in fact, an independent contractor with the ER and CTMF and he did not see a conflict of interest. Ultimately, Fischer-Mangold signed a contract to manage the physician personnel of the emergency room. As with the rest of the multiple factors nationally and locally that were swirling and progressing around the times of the 1970s, emergency medicine, as a specialty, was a new phenomenon. It was not until two years after the contract with Fisher-Mangold was made, that the American Board of Medical Specialties granted the long-sought recognition to emergency medicine as a separate specialty. Dr. Mangold, the immediate past president of the American College of Emergency Physicians, (ACEP) in 1979, had been a champion of that effort.

Dr. Blewett became the director of the physician emergency services at Brackenridge ER and Fischer-Mangold retained the contract for the emergency room until 1995. At that time the management of Brackenridge Hospital was leased to the Seton Network. Em-Care, which was managing the emergency rooms at the Seton Hospitals, acquired the contract. Most of the core physicians in 1977 continued to work in the ER under contract with Fischer-Mangold until the contract changed to Em-care.[38]

One of those core doctors, Dr. Ken Sherman, completed his internship at Brackenridge and rotated on the surgical service at the same time I was covering the orthopedic clinical service. He was an enthusiastic intern and came to the orthopedic clinic regularly. He also came to several of the surgical cases with which I was involved. He was able to assist me in surgery, sew up some wounds, set a fractured arm, make rounds, and, as he said some years later, "have a lot of fun with good learning." He eventually worked in the emergency room eight years. In the early 1980s Dr. Blewett left Brackenridge, along with Dr. Connell and Dr. Boch to started the emergency medicine group at St. David's, mentioned earlier. Dr. Sherman started working part time at St. David's in 1984. Fisher-Mangold looked upon that as a conflict of interest so, by mutual consent, he left Brackenridge for full time coverage at St. David's. Seton hospital had opened its emergency room in 1975 and St. David's was just getting their ER going in the early 1980's. Eventually Dr. Sherman moved his practice to Elgin, Texas and opened a general practice, where he has continued for thirty years.

Dr. Sherman recalls one of his more traumatic and instructive experiences as an intern caring for an orthopedic patient of Dr. Tim Lowry. Dr. Sherman responded to an emergency code call to check on a patient, whom the nurses thought was not breathing. He raced to the room and was contemplating an endotracheal airway when Dr. Lowry, who must have been nearby, walked into the room. Dr. Lowry went to the patient's bedside, quickly evaluated the situation, re-positioned the patient's head with a pillow and the patient promptly started breathing well. Dr. Lowry said, "sometimes just the simple things are best." Ken was thoroughly impressed and learned a quick lesson.

He also related the story of his third week as an intern. He was notified that a patient from San Marcos was being transferred, pregnant, and in eclampsia with seizures. She was admitted directly to the obstetrics floor and, correctly, as the first treatment, he turned her on her side, which reduced her blood pressure. The experienced nurse that was present said, "I can't believe you are just an intern." This helped his pride and was a balancing experience when compared to the orthopedic patient he saw later with difficulty breathing.[39]

One of our patients in the mid 1970's, was a coed in the emergency room with a broken leg. Small motor scooters had become very popular with students at UT. Unfortunately they don't do well when colliding with solid objects, like the bumper of a car. This patient of mine arrived in the emergency room with an unstable mid tibia and fibula fracture. Treatment at that time had progressed from traction and later casting to the use of an external fixation device. That device involved placing two pins above the fracture and two pins below the fracture through the skin and into the tibial bone. These pins were then clamped into an external frame that would maintain three-dimensional stability. Dr. Sherman assisted with that procedure. The coed, besides being a good sport and pretty tough, was a very pretty blond who garnered some attention on the ward. After a few days, she was up on crutches and walking in the hall. She was discharged home to her parents' house in Houston since she was not going to be able to go to class. Four to five days later she called in a panic. She had maggots in the wounds around her pins. Routine care of the pins involved daily cleaning with hydrogen peroxide. She must have missed a day or two. She was completely freaked out and wanted to know what to do about the maggots. I told her to just clean around the pins with alcohol that would sting a little, kill the maggots, and sterilize the wounds. It turned out she had been sun bathing in the warm Houston weather and flies had laid their eggs in the moist tissue around the pins. I attempted to calm her by saying that maggots had been used for years to clean up wounds and she had just had a good side effect. She went on to uneventful healing and returned to the university.

All of the complexities of management, changing personnel, new emergency room, and interaction with the Emergency Medical Service (EMS), had a significant influence for the training program. Except for a few patients from outlying clinics, the majority of patients managed by the house staff came through the emergency room. Rotation in the emergency room was part of some training rotations. The patients that were admitted to the floors were nearly all initially evaluated in the ER. Over the years, the evaluation of patients was markedly improved by the availability of well-trained emergency medicine doctors, who were well versed in acute care. That evaluation and care became a significant part of intern and resident training. They would be notified from the ER of a potential patient admission early in a patient's care and the trainee would come to the ER to join in that evaluation. From overcrowded care in the hallway location of the emergency room in the 1950's and 1960's to the streamlined, efficient location and management of the new facilities a major step in the care of Austin patients was provided. As time passed and telecommunication was added to the ambulance service, the evaluation of emergency patients became more complex in the field by trained emergency medical technicians. Early treatment also was added to the protocols of the ambulances in the field as knowledge, equipment, and training progressed.

A New Training Program

With the articles of incorporation having been completed in March of 1972 for the Central Texas Medical Foundation, the organization of the training programs was to be quickly initiated. Four services would have full time directors: general surgery, internal medicine, pediatrics and obstetrics/gynecology. A fifth service, family medicine, would be organized within a couple of years. Dr. Pape would remain the early director of medical education, however, his responsibilities would involve coordination of the various training services but would also include his responsibilities in the emergency room. Until 1973 there were still internship rotations in the ER. Dr. Pape, along with Drs. Kirksey, Hood and others, was also involved in training emergency medical technician for the new ambulance service. Dr. Pape remained as medical director until Dr. Earl Matthews was hired in 1975, to cover that position as full time director.

Pediatrics

Dr. Karen Teel was the first to be hired as a program director in the fall of 1972. She was to begin the work of developing a pediatric residency program. She graduated from Baylor University College of Medicine in 1963, and completed her internship and residency at Baylor, including Ben Taub Hospital and Texas Children's Hospital. She then completed a two-year infectious disease fellowship in Houston. Following her training, Dr. Teel worked as a pediatrician for four years, 1968 to 1972, at Bergstrom Air Force Base Hospital and clinics. As she had limited experience in running a program, she depended a great deal on Dr. William (Bill) Daeschner, head of Pediatrics at the Texas Medical Branch in Galveston, who would provide excellent guidance for the new program to develop a curriculum and program evaluation. The program was to be called the Austin Pediatric Education Program (APEP). They arranged a formal affiliation with the department of pediatrics in Galveston that would provide regular faculty, residents and students to rotate to Austin. Subspecialty faculty would provide consultation and eventually come to Austin to develop subspecialty clinics. The program established affiliations with the Austin State Hospital for psychiatric treatment, University of Texas, Austin (UT) Speech and Hearing Center, UT Learning Disabilities Center, Austin Child Guidance Center, Texas State School for the Deaf, Austin Evaluation Center, and the Texas State School for the Blind.

The pediatricians of Austin were uniquely united and supportive of the program. They admitted most of their patients to the new children's wing of the hospital. This was of benefit to the teaching program but was also financially helpful as they were able to maintain a good mix of private patients with the charity patients. There were about 27 community pediatricians involved. Particularly supportive and active on the service were Drs. Ben White, Byron (Phil) Kocen, Clinton Craven, Ron Boern, Miles Sedberry, Cliff Price, and Richard Holt, who came in 1973, and Ellis Gill and David Gamble, who came a year or two later. Arrangements were made for all of the community doctors to provide coverage for the clinics. This had been an ongoing service to the hospital through the years and was strengthened with the new program. Pediatric subspecialty service was provided by a number of doctors who had training in Cardiology, Neurology, Infectious Disease, and Child Development. This was to be supplemented by the faculty from Galveston. Dr. Hector Morales started his general surgery practice and included pediatric surgery. Dr. Abraham Besserman followed as a pediatric general surgeon, Dr. Jacob Kay as a neonatologist in 1974, Dr. James Sharp, a hematologist and oncologist and later Dr. George Sharp as a neonatologist, added to the local expertise. As part of the training program specifically, Dr. Teel developed a weekly Pediatric Conference for the overall house staff, weekly Pediatric Grand Rounds, three times a week teaching rounds with Dr. Teel, monthly clinical pathological conference, and monthly basic science lectures. The attending physicians from the community made daily rounds on their patients. Arrangements were made for the residents to rotate out of the hospital to private pediatric offices for that outpatient experience.

As early as October of 1973 the AMA had approved the application of the program for first and second year residency training. Full recruiting of residents was ongoing in May of 1974 for the class to start in July. In the early days of the program it was clearly a building period, but more and more applicants were attracted to the program and the city.[40,41] By 1975 there were three first year, three second year and one third year resident. One of the first year residents, Dr. Charlotte Ann Weaver, completed the program and remained in Austin for her practice. Dr. Tom Zavaleta, who had completed medical school in 1974 at Albert Einstein University, had his first year internship/residency in San Antonio, then switched to Austin for his second year pediatric residency in 1974-75 and a third year in 1976-77. He practiced pediatrics in Austin for over twenty year. He returned for more training as a family practice resident at Brackenridge in 1998 and in 1999 rotated through our office for a month of orthopedic surgery as part of his training. He then remained in Austin to joint the Austin Regional Clinic. At the time of his pediatric residency, 1974-77, in Austin, the pediatric patients were cared for on the 4th floor of the new Brackenridge tower and the pediatric intensive care unit was still in the red brick building.

Dr. Zavaleta recalled that during his residency there would periodically be a child, who was so ill, that it was felt best to have care handled in Galveston. That meant an ambulance drive to UTMB with the patient and a pediatric resident going along to take care of the child. The ambulance driver seemed to need a little fun diversion on the drive across the flat country of the Coastal Plains. Driving at 80-90 miles per hour, he would turn on his microphone and start making "mooing" sounds to the cows in the nearby fields. The cows would start running to the fence in response, much to the joy of the driver and the resident. There was no more "mooing" after the start of "Star flight" helicopters in 1985.[42]

In those early days of the program, before recruiting started in 1974, the pediatric inpatients were admitted to the old red brick building on the general medicine floor. At that point the trainees were all rotating interns with the addition of students and residents from Galveston. The program was moved to the east end of the fourth floor in the new tower and the nursing care was provided by the general medical nursing pool. Many of those nurses did not have special training in pediatrics. That could be a problem as medication dosages were quite different from adults. Dr. Milton Talbot, a 1946 graduate of Tulane Medical School, moved to Austin in 1971 after an eighteen-year practice in Big Spring, Texas. He and Dr. Teel became very involved in making changes in the department. They created a pediatric intensive care unit on the sixth floor of the new building and moved toward more specialized nursing care on that floor. Eventually they outgrew the bed capacity in the main Brackenridge tower. A new pediatric hospital was planned for the corner of 15th Street and the I-35 access road. This would greatly improve the children's services and space for the teaching program. By the time the new hospital was built in 1988 there were 14-16 residents in the three-year program. In addition to the residents' experience in the hospital, they rotated through private pediatricians' offices throughout the city. This experience was very valuable as this would be the form of most of their work as they established their own office practices following training. As the major contact with patients is in the hospital or hospital clinics in most training programs this office experience is not available to many training programs throughout the country.

When Dr. Teel began her job she noted that there were only two books on pediatrics in the medical library. That, among many other things, would have to be improved. There would continue to be problems in implementing a full time program including maintaining the necessary staff, materials, clinics, and battling with administration (basically the City) about money. In 1977, Dr. Teel left the program for private practice with Drs. Jack Lewis, Dilip Karnik, and Bill Caldwell. Dr. Teel, among many others, had many difficulties with Mr. Brown, the administrator. This was just before Mr. Spurk became acting administrator. Dr. Jim Sharpe followed Dr. Teel and became the acting director of the teaching program and remained in that position for almost two years. He inherited a program that still had some difficulties. It was during that time that there was a site visitation by the residency accreditation committee, and because of several deficiencies, including the lack of a dedicated ambulatory care service, the program was put on probation. This adversely affected the recruiting of residents, since potential recruits had to be told the program was on probation. Dr. Sharpe, along with the help of Dr. Dykes Cordell, a pediatric cardiologist, worked hard and got the program off probation and back on course by 1980. Funding was obtained for an ambulatory care director. Dr. Anthony (Toni) Kimbrough was hired by CTMF for the position. He was a UTMB graduate who did his pediatric training in San Antonio. He set up outpatient clinics at the East Austin Health Clinics and set up a more standard program. Eventually, Dr. Kimbrough wound up doing more managing of the entire pediatric program as Dr. Cordell was absent a lot, perhaps with some health problems. Dr. Cordell resigned in about 1981 and Dr. Kimbrough became the acting director while the search for a full time director was completed.[40]

In 1982 Dr. George A. Edwards was hired for the positions of director of the pediatric program. A graduate of Rice University and Baylor Medical School, he had done his pediatric residency at Baylor. He became interested in nephrology and did a fellowship in that area, including a stint in Los Angeles, studying creatinine clearance and glomerulular filtration. He then joined a pediatric practice in North Carolina for five years. His wife, Marci, was interested in persuing a PhD. The University of Texas in Austin was attractive and, as the job in Austin for pediatric director opened up, they moved to Austin in June, 1983. At that time, Dr. Earl Matthews was the director of medical education in Austin. The pediatric department was on the fourth floor of the new hospital tower and there were twelve residents in the program. The neonatal intensive care unit (NICU) still had a presence in the old red brick building, quite a distance from the main pediatric unit, and the ambulatory care clinic was in East Austin. In January of 1983, Dr. Khadayer Bahranmi was the resident on call. When he came in to round on the NICU he found that the pipes had frozen and broken in the new Brackenridge building, the NICU had four inches of water on the floor, and all of the patients needed to be moved to another area. The patients were moved to the post operative recovery room in the new building where they remained until the new ICU was completed on the second floor off the circular drive at the main entrance of the building.

When taking over the pediatric program, Dr. Edwards had a moderate amount of experience in administration of a program, having been involved in programs in Houston, Los Angeles and North Carolina. However he did not have direct hands on administrative experience. He also did not have much experience with the American College of Graduate Medical Education (ACGME), the accrediting body for resident training programs. He had arrived in June and there was another ACGME site visit in September 1983. The program did not do well with that review as the review panel felt the program had insufficient sub-specialty coverage and emergency medicine. The determination was appealed and the review panel revised the emergency medicine determination to passing, but sustained the specialty coverage criticism. That kept the program on probation, contributing to the problems with recruitment for a second time. Arrangements were made with the pediatric programs in Galveston and Houston for more specialty coverage. The contribution by the University of Texas Medical Branch over the years to several of the programs in Austin, but particularly the pediatrics program, was invaluable. With specialty coverage from Galveston and Houston in place, the ACGME site visit in 1987 went well, and the program was taken off probation. After three years on probation there were a handful of U. S. graduates and a number of foreign medical graduates in the program. The perception that the foreign graduates were not as strong as US graduates resulted in additional recruiting problems. It is noted that many of the foreign graduates were bright students. Dr. Khadayer Bahrami, the resident who discovered the water in the NICU, went on to do a neonatology fellowship and eventually worked in the Children's National Medical Center using extra-corporeal membrane oxygenation for children with under developed lung capacity. Another resident, Jesus Eric Pena went on to do a fellowship in neurology and later became the director at Vanderbilt for the pediatric program. Our Austin program regained its good standing with the ACGME and has been accredited continuously since 1987.

In the mid 1980's, a major step forward was made with the building of the new Children's Hospital on the corner of 15th and I-35. This had been the dream of Dr. Talbot and Dr. Teel. The old red brick building that had occupied that space had been torn down in the late 1970's.

In the mid 1980's a system of payment for hospital care under Medicare and Medicaid was created whereby reimbursement for hospital stays would be based on various diagnosis related groups (DRGs). Thus a specific diagnosis was used to determine the payment for hospital treatment for that diagnosis. This lump sum payment varied as to how completely the cost of hospital care was covered. As it did not take into consideration the total amount of work done, it was generally accepted that this system would adversely affect payment for services. For some reason, rehabilitation medicine and pediatric care were excluded from payment under DRGs. That payments system provided a psychological support and also a financial support for these services. As a result, a plethora of rehabilitation hospitals were built in the 1980's. It was also sufficient incentive for the City of Austin to invest in a new Pediatric Hospital. The new Children's Hospital of Austin was completed in 1988. With the successful accreditation of the program in 1987 and the new hospital in 1988 the recruiting efforts became much more successful. By the early 1990's the majority of the residents were graduates of American medical schools and filling the programs slots did not depend on foreign medical students. In the years 1990 to 1992 there were fifteen to sixteen residents with one chief resident. By 1995 there were 20 residents including the chief resident.

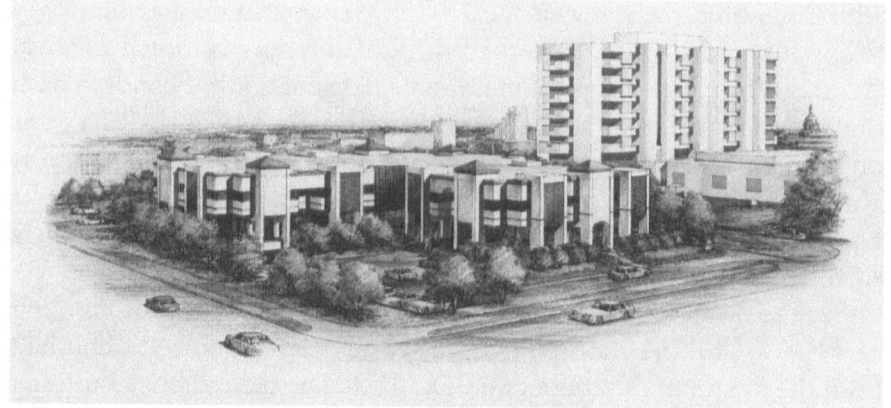

Artist's rendition of Children's Hospital on the corner of 15th and IH-35 with Brackenridge Hospital in background. (with permission, Austin History Center, Austin Public Library.

By the late 1990's and early 2000's the Austin Pediatric hospital on the corner of 15th and I-35 was quite successful, in large part due to the support of the local pediatricians who admitted most of their patients at that facility. Because of the positive contribution of private paying patients, no inclusion in the DRGs reimbursement program, and Children's Health Insurance Program (CHIP) (for children in families who earned too much for Medicaid eligibility and not enough for insurance), the hospital became very successful and began to outgrow its space and beds. Because it was located next to Brackenridge on a limited amount of ground and had structural limitations to making the building taller, the idea of creating an entirely new hospital in a new location became attractive.

In 1995 the management of Brackenridge hospital had become much more burdensome for the City. The training program had become much more complex and difficult for the Central Texas Medial Foundation to fund and manage. Between 1990 and 1998 the budget for the training program had grown from about $2 million to $7-8 million. In the class of 1995 there were approximately 71 residents in all of the programs, including six transitional interns.

At this time there was a hotbed of activity with formation of Health Maintenance Organizations (HMOs). To maintain favorable relationships with these HMOs, a hospital had to provide a broad range of services. Under the direction of Mr. Barnett, CEO, Seton became strongly interested in developing a hospital network to provide a broader geographic service area. A contract with the city would expand Seton's network, adding Brackenridge, the trauma center, and for pennies on the dollar, would put them in the driver's seat of the pediatric hospital, adding a huge advantage in dealing with HMOs. It would have cost millions to develop a strong pediatric service at Seton as a separate facility from Children's and it was unpredictable whether the pediatric community would support a separate facility. Not only was the pediatric hospital not under the restrictive DRG payment arrangement but the neonatal intensive care unit (NICU) was a very high income center. Seton would find a 'bird nest on the ground" with such a contract.

The Seton Healthcare Network signed a management contract with the City to run Brackenridge in 1995. Seton became interested in the training program and in 1998 negotiations between CTMF and Seton resulted in the sale of the training program to Seton. Over the next 10 years, Seton investigated and developed a plan to build a new children's hospital. Their initiative and funding, with community support, and money from the Dell Foundation led to the construction of an entirely new facility on the old Mueller Airport site east of IH 35.

An interesting event gave a boost to this project coming to fruition. Seton was comfortable with managing the existing children's hospital on 15th street. They did not see the necessity of building a new facility beyond what they had. Several doctors, including Drs. Pat Connolly, George Edwards, Richard Holt, Robert Schlechter, and others held a news conference on the steps of the court house to publicize their position on the need for a new and larger pediatric hospital. It is felt that this event got Mr. Barnett, CEO of the Seton Network, more informed about the pediatricians position. That event may have also resulted in donation of land for a children's hospital at the Mueller tract, the prior airport site. It also provided information to the public and impetus to the Dell Foundation to become involved.

The Seton Hospital System is now the primary owner of the new hospital. The new Dell Children's Medical Center of Central Texas was completed in July of 2007. The neonatal intensive care unit was moved to the new building as the initial building occupant. The rest of the patients were moved in one day by a series of ambulances to the Children's center with no complications. The current facility has a full complement of pediatric subspecialty departments, from Allergy to Pharmacy, with the exception of a burn unit and a transplant program.[43]

With the move away from the Brackenridge campus there was some loss of institutional memory. Mr. Bob Bonar, an administrator at Brackenridge, was very involved in developing and implementing plans for the new hospital but he had since left the institution. As Seton evolved in its management of Brackenridge, the training program, and the new Children's Hospital, a lot of bureaucracy has developed in the management processes. Sister Theresa, the long-standing heart of Seton, had retired and the emotional make up was significantly changed. This is perhaps inherent in organizations as they become larger, particularly those required to dance to the drum of multiple state and federal rules and regulations. Many employee's job descriptions involve creating paper work, fulfilling regulation requirements, collecting numbers for statistical analysis, changing procedures to follow the rules, and moving from a people friendly community to a bureaucratic system that seems less warm. There are many reasons to believe that there will be better patient outcomes but it is more difficult to feel those results.

There is definitely room in the new system for creating new ideas and programs. One new program, a Child Development Abuse consultation service, is working to provide better care for a segment of children that were not well served in the past. Ten years earlier the social workers had noted there was a lot of inconsistency in the care of abused children. With this service there would be an accumulation of resources to allow the community to rally around these children and improve the treatment of those problems. In 2011 additional grant money was obtained to augment this program. A second program supported by a 2011 grant would be to establish a "Failure to Thrive Clinic" with additional support services. These initiatives would add to the experience for training residents who would encounter these problems in their own community practices.[43]

Another physician who came to Austin in July, 1973 would make a significant contribution to the program as his practice evolved. Dr. Richard Holt went to medical school in Galveston and then went to Duke University for a pediatric internship and residency. As it became apparent at Duke that he had had a great deal of practical experience in medical school, he was assigned to the neonatal intensive care unit. He found the program very interesting and challenging but highly academic and competitive. His interest, however, was in general pediatrics, so, after a year at Duke, he returned to Galveston to complete his final two years. He did some "locum tenens" work with Dr. Clinton Cravens in Austin during his training. That led to him to join the practice with Drs. Cravens, Jack Kidd, Phil Kocen, and replacing Dr. Pat Cato who had become ill. They maintained a general pediatric practice until 1988, when they joined the Austin Diagnostic Clinic. As the subspecialty of hospitalists for adult care had becoming more of a trend, Dr. Holt began to explore the possibility of becoming a hospitalist for the pediatric community. The pediatric community had remained very supportive of the Children's hospital and they were likely to be supportive of this concept. He talked about this with his partners and they were very much in favor of the idea. They offered to supplement his salary as he got his practice started, knowing it might be slow at first. In 1993 he began the switch in his practice. He negotiated a contract with UTMB for teaching, a contract with Seton to be the medical director, and gained the support of many community pediatricians. All of the Austin Diagnostic Clinics doctors sent their patients to him. Some other pediatricians sent him patients from time to time. The service became so convenient for them since they would no longer have to go to the hospital to make rounds, he received patients from other community pediatricians. Dr. Karen Teel, founder of the training program, made a commitment and stated she was sending all of her patients to Dr. Holt. She told him, "I am going to send all of my patients to you as long as you take care of them as well as I do." That changed the complexion of the service for, from that time on, most admissions were made to his service. This was a bit of a natural move since the pediatric community had been so supportive of the program at Brackenridge for so many years. After about two years, almost all patients referred to the hospital were cared for by Dr. Holt (with the exception of patients from a large multispecialty clinic, Austin Regional Clinic). With time he became more and more involved with the teaching program as he was at the hospital taking care of the patients who would also become teaching patients for the resident staff. In 1995, he and Dr. Maria Forbes, a faculty member for ambulatory care, joined forces to increase the inpatient care available. As part of his involvement with the teaching program, he made trips to the Cleveland Clinic and to Cook County to observe how those programs were run.

Not only did the community support the program but the program director, Dr. George Edwards, was very interested in Dr. Holt's presence as a full time pediatric hospitalist. This pediatric hospitalist program evolved from daily inpatient care to twenty-four hour care when they moved to the new Dell Children's Hospital. And by 2015, it had grown to thirty doctors and had demonstrated a better level of patient care and a higher nurse retention rate.[44]

The standard approach to patient's hospital admissions in teaching institutions in Austin and across the country has been their assignment of patients to a particular service, primarily dependent on their status as a paying or charity case. The patients who were referred in by Dr. Holt's former office at Austin Diagnostic Clinic, or other private physician's offices, generally had insurance and were able to pay for their private care. They would be assigned to one service. With evolution, that became Dr. Holt's service with the assistance of the residents. Patients referred in from city and county clinics or the emergency room, were generally less well funded or had no funds at all. The unfunded patients were routinely assigned to another service in the care of the residents in the training program and their supervisors.

With progression of care, Dr. Edwards developed the concept that there should be one service with a uniform approach for all patients. This would eliminate the two-service system and the implication that there were, medically, two levels of care. By the mid 1990's, all pediatric patients were admitted to a single service with no "means" testing. This meant that all patients, whether covered by private insurance, Medicaid, CHIP, MAP (City Medical Assisted Program for hospital care), Aid to Families with Dependent Children (AFDC), or cases from outside the county, were cared for with no distinction between service assignment. This system of care has been facilitated by the fact that most children in Texas have some funding from one of the above programs. It is unusual to have a child for whom no funding is available or for whom none can be arranged. As adult funding is less complete it is more difficult to reproduce this model in adult hospital care.

Another program that became critical to pediatric care in Austin was the addition of neonatal intensive care. Dr. Holt had considered that specialty as a possible avenue of practice in his early years. He had visited with Dr. Jacob Kay in Dallas to discuss issues in that specialty. Dr. Kay put it simply. He was single with no family that would compete with his time and he "spent his life in the hospital." As Richard had a family, Dr. Kay did not feel that newborn intensive care was a reasonable fit for him or most physicians. Dr. Holt took that advice and did not continue in pursuit of that subspecialty. In the late 1970s, Dr. Clinton Craven was involved in raising funds to try to get a neonatologist to come to Austin. Dr. Kay, to whom Dr. Holt had talked earlier, was ultimately recruited to Austin. He, with the later additions of Dr. George Sharp, contributed significantly to pediatric care and teaching in Austin, both at Brackenridge and at St. David's. Although St. David's is a private hospital, it takes care of many new mothers who are funded by Medicaid. The doctors at St. David's deliver a huge number of infants whose mothers are poorly funded and not well motivated to prenatal care. As a consequence, they have a disproportionate number of premature or small babies or have other conditions that require neonatal intensive care. The availability of neonatal care has added enormously to the community at St. David's as well as to the training program at Children's hospital.[43,44]

And so, the pediatric program, the first truly organized under the Travis County Medical Foundation and, arguably, the best supported by the community doctors, has continued to grow, adding beds, hospitals, doctors and services to the benefit of the residents in training and the community in general.

Internal Medicine

There are not many details about some of the early trainees listed in this program. There was no formal program in the 1950's. The records indicate that Dr. Charles E. Davis was in Austin from July 1, 1950 to October 16, 1950 as a medicine and pediatric resident. He then left for military leave of absence. Dr. Rafael S. Villareal was a rotating intern from July 1950 to the end of December 1950 and then is listed in medicine and pediatrics from January 1951 to June 1952 (18 months). Although there are other residents listed from the mid 1950's to 1973, none are specifically identified as internal medicine residents.

From the very early days of CTMF, the Internal Medicine section had co-directors Drs. Jack Moncreif and Jonathan Decherd, who were board certified internal medicine specialists, with subspecialties in nephrology. Both were graduates of UTMB. With active practices of their own and much of it centered in Brackenridge, they decided to take on the program and develop the rotations, conferences, lectures and patient care that would be required. Dr. Moncrief arrived in Austin in 1968 and Dr. Decherd in 1971. As nephrologists, both were very involved in the early kidney program at Brackenridge. Dr. Moncrief and Dr. Maurice Hood were instrumental in the first kidney transplant in central Texas in January, 1972. Many of their patients were also under the care of cardiothoracic and vascular surgeons Drs. Kirksey, Hood, Calhoon, Arnold, and Tate, since many of them had cardiac problems as well as kidney disease or would require surgery. Dr. Moncrief and later Dr. Decherd mentored students rotating as externs from Galveston in nephrology. Dr. John Boyd was one of those externs who became interested in doing his internship here in 1972. Dr. Moncrief and Dr. Dechard had discussed creating an internal medicine residency since they already had externs rotating through their service. With CTMF forming an overall structure, they volunteered to take on the new program as it was being developed under CTMF. They had no support staff or secretarial help and they used their office staff at Austin Diagnostic Clinic for letters and paper work. Their trainees at that point were interns, externs and some residents rotating up from Galveston. In 1974 one resident was based at Brackenridge. By 1975, when CTMF hired Dr. Tim Stevens as full time medical director for the internal medicine department, there were five flexible interns, five first-year, four second-year and one third-year resident in internal medicine. One of the interns, Charlie Moore, went on through the program and stayed in Austin. Dr. Dan Finch, one of the second-year residents stayed in Austin after completing his training.[45]

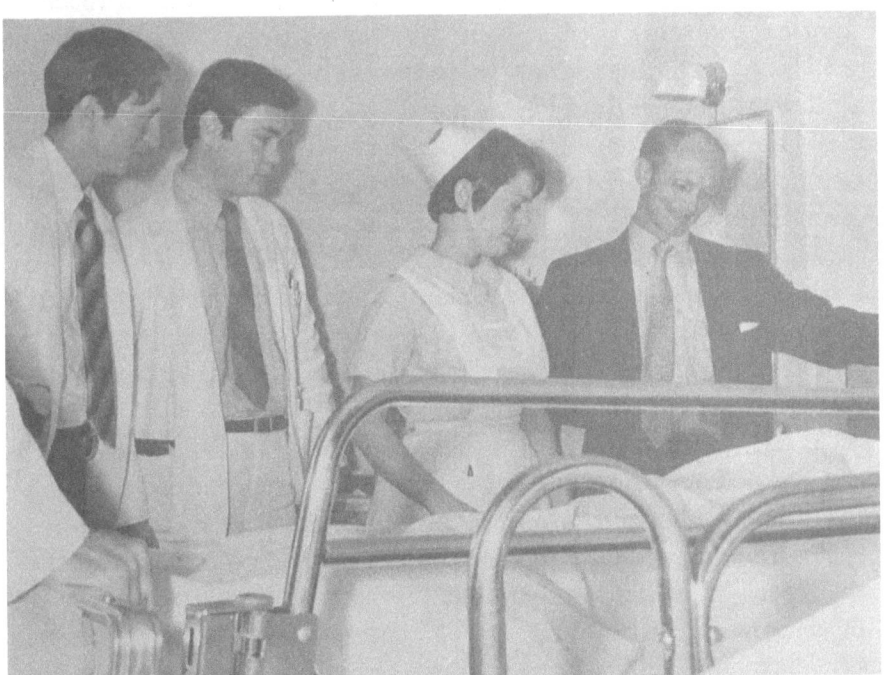

Dr. Jack Moncrief (far right) mentoring interns and students in the late 1960's. Dr. Ken Teafel intern on left.

The program operated a large inpatient service at Brackenridge, consisting primarily of patient who came to the ER without a private doctor (non-preference patients) and charity patients from various clinics. City Medical Assistance Program (MAP) patients from the Sabine clinic next to the hospital and three Health and Human Services clinics in south and east Austin were also served through the internal medicine department. Most of these patients were admitted through the emergency room. As with the other services, the emergency room was covered by internists on a rotating basis so that the patients were admitted under their names but co-managed by the teaching service. There was an evolution of specialty care and management of the clinics. There had been diabetic clinic, tuberculosis, allergy, and general medicine clinics under the eye of Dr. Lang Holland as far back as the 1940's. He was still running the diabetic clinic as late as 1969. Dr. Bob Morrison was an early tuberculosis and pulmonary specialist and ran the tuberculosis clinic as early as 1950. Dr. Jack Schneider, an urologist, did his residency at the Mayo Clinic. Urology residents studied the surgical approach to urological problems but also were involved with the medical issues of the kidneys, including kidney disease and kidney failure. There were no nephrologists at the time Dr. Schneider arrived in Austin, so he spent many hours at Brackenridge doing urology. He was also involved in the care of patients with kidney failure in conjunction with the internists.[46] As more subspecialists opened practices in Austin, they expanded and supervised the various clinics. As noted earlier, Dr. Felger came in 1968 and was involved in the subspecialty of gastroenterology. Although his practice was with the Austin Diagnostic Clinic, the center of his activities and his great interest were at Brackenridge where he admitted most of his patients.[33]

As part of the training program being set up in 1972, the trainees were "farmed out" to various private practice offices for experience. Not only did they follow Dr. Moncreif and Dr. Decherd, they spent time in general internal medicine, gastroenterology, diabetes mellitus care, and other specialist's offices. Of course, taking care of sick patients in the hospital was crucial but their future practices would be in offices as well as the hospital, so this office experience was important.

Dr. Stevens noted that Dr. Moncreif reviewed the records of many Brackenridge patients in the adult medical clinic and divided them up according to their predominant medical subspecialty problem. He then assigned patients and physician to subspecialty clinics and in a sense, created a primary care environment for the patients. Dr. Stevens established weekly primary care clinics for the residents, creating these clinics using patient in the subspecialty clinics, and changing the subspecialty clinics to become more consultation clinics.

Dr. Stevens followed Dr. Moncreif and Dr. Dechard as director of internal medicine. He was trained as an internist with a subspecialty in cardiology. He would be involved in managing conferences and grand rounds, and supervising resident while maintaining a busy practice running the cardiac catheter laboratory. Dr. Stevens was in practice by himself, he did not have a lot of cross coverage for his patients. He managed the call schedule, the resident rotations, community staff involvement and recruiting of new residents each year

In 1975 the CTMF hired Dr. Earl Matthews as the director of medical education and Dr. Tim Stevens as head of internal medicine. Dr. Matthews had completed an internal medicine residency and then an infectious disease subspecialty in San Antonio. It would be his responsibility to coordinate the various services, assist with achieving and maintaining accreditation of each service, coordinate any cross over activities, assist with conferences, arrange for outside consultants and resources, and communicate with CTMF. Funding was to be a continuous battle, as taking care of indigent patients and paying for interns and residents was definitely not a money-making business. Dr. Matthews remained in that position until 1997 when funding problems caused him to seek other opportunities. During his tenure he consulted in infectious disease at Brackenridge as well as other hospitals in Austin.[47]

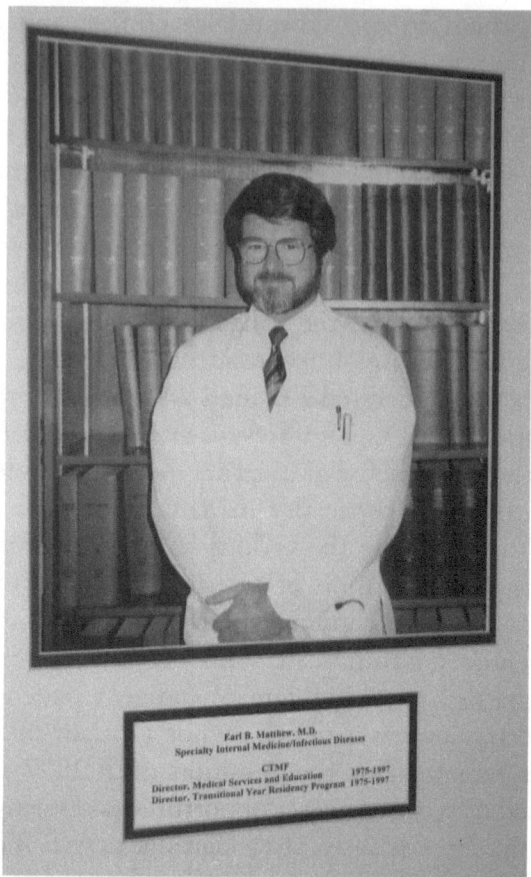

Dr. Earl Matthews, first Medical director of
the CTMF program, 1975-1998.

There had been a medical staff office with secretaries and management personnel as early as the early 1970s but this would grow as the programs became bigger and more complicated. In the 1975-76 year there were five transitional interns, five first year, four second year and one third year internal medicine trainee in addition to three pathology residents, seven pediatric residents, five flexible interns, ten family practice residents, and the surgery residents from St. Joseph's in Houston. This resulted in forty house staff to be managed under the umbrella of the training program managed by Dr. Matthews. By the 1979-80 year there were just over fifty house staff.

Dr. Tim Stevens wrote a letter some years later to Dr. Fleeger noting the many doctors who volunteered their time at Brackenridge with the teaching program and the clinics. In cardiology were Drs. Robert Anderson, Bill McCarron, George Lowe, Bert Joseph, Archie Robinson, Michael Rotman, and Tom Runge. The dermatologist was Sam Thompson. In endocrinology were Drs. Ross Chiles, Terry Collier, Henry Renfert, and Joe Volpe. The gastroenterologists were Drs. Fred Bieberdorf, Rambie Briggs, Charlie Felger, Tom McHorse, and George Kitzmiller. Contributing in hematology and oncology were Drs. Robert Kerr, Doug Terry, Dennis Welch, Dudly Youman, and John Sandbach. Dr. Earl Matthews as director of the training program also provided expertise in infectious disease. The nephrologist included Drs. Jonathan Decherd, Jack Moncrief, Gerald Beathard and Jim Lindley. Drs. Everett Heinze, Harold Skaggs, and Jerry Tindel were the neurologist involved. The pulmonologist were Drs. Robert Emerson, George Handley, Robert Morrison (going back many years), and Jim Lindsey. Finally the rheumatologists were Drs. Jim Crout, Homer Goehrs, and Marshall Sack.

Dr. Lysbeth (Beth) Miller graduated from the University of Texas at San Antonio in 1979, followed by her internal medicine residency at the University of North Carolina. In 1983 she came to Austin where her husband had a job. After three years with the Austin Regional Clinic she then joined the Austin Diagnostic Clinic for a year. She was not very busy during the day but was covered up with night work in the ER. As the younger doctor in that practice, she needed to establish her own patients, but the night call was quite taxing. With young children at home that was not a very satisfactory schedule. She was involved at Brackenridge, as were other community doctors, taking her one-month rotations in the ER, admitting patients and rounding with the residents. As she found private practice rather tame compared to work at Brackenridge and the night call rather onerous, when an opening for an assistant to Dr. Stevens opened in 1987, she applied and was hired. She said she pushed rather hard to get the job. During her first three months on the job she found great opportunities for strengthening the teaching program. The conferences were limping along. The staff doctors were only making rounds three times a week with the residents. When she noted one of the residents reading from Harrison's Textbook of Internal Medicine, a very outdated book, she knew she could make a differnce. Dr. Stevens was so busy in the catheter laboratory that supervision was insufficient. The general internal medicine clinic was basically unsupervised although sub-specialty support was very good in the specialized clinics as the community doctors were providing regular support. What was most alarming was that the mortality rate for patients on the floor was too high. By instituting stronger resident supervision, more regular bedside rounds, intensive care unit treatment protocols, and other initiatives, she was able to drastically reduce the mortality rate for patients. By augmenting the mortality and morbidity conference, marked improvement in treatment and patient support was achieved. She also learned, by going to national medical director conferences that many changes would have to be made to bring the training up to an appropriate level and consistent with other programs.

Dr. Miller also noted that, although the numbers of recruited doctors for resident positions was good, the strength of the applicants could have been better. Austin was a popular place to come but the program needed to be strengthened so that stronger applicants would be available. The major concern revolved around foreign medical graduates as residents. These residents required added time to be integrated into the American system of medical treatment, history and physical record keeping, interaction with nursing, and the hospital in general. This took time away from the primary goal of medical teaching.

There are always multiple factors that will affect a complicated program such as medical care and teaching. Money was always an issue. With the increased number of residents and patients the staff needed also to be increased. The budget for all the training programs grew from around $3 million in the early 1980's to $15 million around 1990. The money came from insurance for a few patients; Medicare, with its complexities for direct patient care; supplements for training; and billing by the staff and consultants to insurance companies, when available. To obtain appropriate reimbursement for patient care by the staff doctors when the residents were also taking care of patients, Medicare and Medicaid had much more stringent requirements. As of 1988, attending doctors had to make more detailed notes in the patient's charts to document staff visits. That responsibility had not been necessary in the past. This required much more time on the part of the teaching staff, including involved community doctors. This was true nation wide. The budgeting process was complicated by the costs, the billed amounts, the actual collections and the known or anticipated "write downs" of non-paying patients and insurance variables. It is one thing to deal with those problems when a hospital day costs $50 or less; but with the vast changes in cost, accounting and various payment sources (Medicare, Medicaid, MAP, Disproportionate share, City of Austin, and occasional insurance), keeping track of the process became difficult. It was particularly difficult for the City Council to understand these numbers as they had very little understanding of a training program and its contribution to the community. It was just another of the many expenses items on the City's budget. During the period from 1975 to 1990 there were six different mayors and many changes in the council make up, so learning the needs and processes was difficult. I'm sure that Brackenridge and the training program were not at the top of the list of the many issues before the council: rapid city growth; traffic; Save Our Springs initiative; protection of the Edwards Aquifer; beautification of the shores of Lady Bird Lake; preservation of historic sites; and the support of the growing music industry. In a system that required the hospital administrator to actually go to the City Council chamber, sit through the meeting to wait his turn, and finally be able to present his request, one can infer a very limited priority level. In the City's defense, they had supported the city hospital for over a century, when most community hospitals were supported by county governments.

Dr. Miller has remained medical director to the present. She has weathered the budgets under the City and the various City managers and assistants. Around 1990 the city budget planner forgot to include an accounting for uninsured patients who would be seen but would not pay anything for their care. There was some scrambling to make adjustment for this in the budget. In 1995, the Seton Hospital System contracted with the City to take over management of Brackenridge under a long-term contract. In 1998 the training program management was transferred from CTMF to Seton, as the financial resources of the medical society were insufficient to continue that management and back up any shortfall in the budget.

In the first few months of the Seton contract Dr. Miller realized that Seton had no real concept of how to deal with a training program. It seemed reasonable that services other than internal medicine would have the same concerns. In their contract with the City, Seton had the responsibility of providing care to indigent patients as the hospital had done since the 1890's. After some deliberation, it appeared that, even with the complexities of managing the training program, retaining that program and all of the care that it could provide would be the least expensive way to make sure that indigent care would continue uninterrupted. In the year 2000, in an effort to capitalize on Austin and Central Texas as an attractive place to join a residency program, the name was changed from CTMF to the Austin Medical Education Program (AMEP).

Dr. Earl Matthews continued to be the Medical Director of all of the various services. With the new management by Seton there was an additional level of bureaucracy and stress added to the system. Dr. Matthews decided, about that time, to "leave for greener pastures." He moved to Corpus Christi to advance his infectious disease practice.[47]

In an effort to enhance the management of the program, Seton reached out to gather more resources. Seton sought additional help to deal with the training program that required management of faculty personnel, a large number of residents, interns and medical students, funding complications with indigent care, and proper accreditation with the Accreditation Council for Graduate Medical Education (ACGME). The University of Texas Medical branch had been our helpmate in obstetrics and gynecology since the 1950's. They had provided specialty care and consultants and had staffed subspecialty clinics in Pediatrics since the early 1970's as that program was established under CTMF.

Beth Miller, as director of the Internal Medicine program, was particularly interested in a relationship with UTMB. By 2003 an agreement with UTMB was completed whereby they would assist with many administrative duties and would even be involved in paying the salaries of the residents, although there was a significant money exchange between Seton and UTMB. The arrangement was an excellent move for the Internal Medicine program as they were able to increase the number of medicine residents to 14 positions and increase the number of patients to around 100 on the inpatient service. This arrangement also benefited UTMB as they sent a number of third year students to Austin for clerkships in medicine, pediatrics, surgery and obstetrics.

The relationship with UTMB was to last until 2008 when multiple complications resulted in a decision by UTMB to terminate the relationship. The faculty at Galveston was very concerned about loosing the medical school on the island and hurricane Ike severely exacerbated that concern by destroying much of their campus. The Austin program had to seek another partner for management of the training programs. That was found with the University of Texas Southwestern Medial School in Dallas. In 2009 UT Southwestern assumed the sponsorship of the program at Brackenridge. They did not supply faculty personnel but provided another Designated Institutional Officer for accreditation management and overall supervision of the programs.

Over the period of the next 6 years, the positions for residents grew to 47 and the faculty grew as well. The faculty included sixteen hospitalists, 3 endocrinologists, three infectious disease specialists and three hematologist/oncologists. Funding from the Texas Higher Education Coordinating Board has, in part, made this possible. The Texas Higher Education Coordination Board has the responsibility for promoting access, affordability, quality, success and cost efficiency in the state's institutions of higher education. There were three independent faculty positions for gastroenterology but that arrangement was eventually scrapped and a contract with the Austin Gastroenterology group was written. Seton was the managing entity relative to establishing the various specialties and faculty. Even with the number of faculty, on such a busy service, keeping the residents in contact with their mentors is sometimes difficult.[48]

One of the oversight elements that has kept the program headed in the right direction is the American Council on Graduate Medical Education (ACGME). In addition to the periodic major visitation surveys of the program, a yearly resident and faculty survey has provided information on the effectiveness of the program. In response to some survey results, programs across the country may have had to provide additional information and paperwork to the Council. The Austin program has done very well in recent years and has not had adverse survey reports from residents and faculty with which they have had to deal. Possibly, as the result of that good record and with the program coming under the umbrella of the new UT Austin Dell Medical School in December of 2014, it is likely that the number of resident positions will increase to sixty-three over the next few years.

In spite of the excitement with the formation of the new medical school, mundane elements of running a program take additional time. One significant problem is dealing with physicians that are hired as employees. Keeping them well motivated is an element of concern. Entering into that equation has been the introduction of electronic medical records. A quagmire of clumsy programs has been produced by the software industry to try to satisfy the many different ideas about how to gather and categorize information. In my experience, reviewing thousands of records in the past ten years for Workers Compensation cases, these electronic medical records are fairly good about listing the patients past history of medical treatment and medications. They are really terrible when recording the nuances of a current medical history. They list things well but leave out all of the thinking and evaluation process used by the physician to truly interpret that historical information. Since the Federal Government is heavily into collecting data and trying to maintain as much control as possible, these electronic medical records are exhausting to complete on a daily basis. This has added time to record keeping both in the clinics and on the hospital floors. Thus, the staff and residents are encountering a higher level of frustration and fatigue, resulting in "burn out," as compared to prior years. It remains to be seen how this will affect the program and the staff through the next several years.

Incorporation of the internal medicine program into the Dell Medical School has resulted in new positions for the staff. Dr. Miller is now an associate professor and director of the internal medicine residency program. Dr. Michael Pignone has been recently named as the inaugural chair of the Department of Internal Medicine. Most of the faculty members are now assistant professors but there are a significant number of volunteer clinical faculty that keep the program active and bring the total number of instructors to around ninety.[48]

Surgery Department

The interns that came to Brackenridge through the years routinely rotated through the general surgery area from the beginning. The second trainee, Dr. Claude Martin, did his internship in Galveston and came to Austin primarily to study surgery. He spent most of that year with the general surgeons and would, thus, be considered a surgical resident. So for the first thirty-eight years the surgeons supported the rotating interns who would spend time in surgery, as well as medicine, pediatrics and obstetrics/gynecology. They would spend a one-month rotation in the emergency room and various other services as time allowed. Surgery was not exclusively general surgery but would include ear, nose and throat, orthopedics, and the other subspecialties.

In 1950, Dr. Kenneth Reidland is listed as chief surgery resident. In that time period surgical residency programs were very hierarchical, in that only one resident was chosen to be chief resident from a program of four or more fourth year positions. I would assume that Dr. Reidland was not selected to be chief resident in the program where he did most of his training and that he came to Brackenridge to benefit from a year as chief. In that year also Dr. Porfior Diaz is listed as a surgical resident. He is not listed the next year. Mary Mika from the residency training office, provided me with lists of the trainees for each year covering seventy-five years. She did not have details of all of the residents so we do not know the history of all of these trainees' prior programs.

Dr. Bernard L. Wellett is listed as a surgery resident for only the years 1953-54. There is a chief surgical resident, Dr. M.S. Madison for 1954-55 and then another chief, Dr. Arthur A. McMurray in 1955-56. It as assumed that these residents came here to have the experience of a year as chief that they did not get elsewhere.

Dr. Leonard Coleman from the Navasota Medical Clinic was a general surgery resident in 1958-59. I would assume that he was in practice there and came to Brackenridge to gain additional experience to supplement the medical staff experience at that clinic. The records show that he was there for one year. Dr. Anthony Manoli came as a second year resident in 1960-61, most likely as a surgery resident, as he stayed to complete his third year in 1962. Dr. Bob Pape, having completed his internship in 1956-57, returned for his first year of surgical residency in 1961 and was there through 1963 when he became the medical director. There are several residents listed in the house staff during the early to mid 1960's, but their departments are not listed. In 1964-65, Dr. J. Fred Kramer was listed as chief surgical resident. It is assumed that he transferred from another program to complete that year of residency. Dr. Franklin C Harmon must have come as a third year in 1964 and then stayed as chief resident through 1966. Dr. Robert Tate, came from the military to do his internship in 1962-63 and then returned for his first year surgery residency in 1965; he is recorded as a third year in 1967-68. He later went on to a cardiovascular program before returning to Austin to practice. I believe it is indicative of the limited organization of the residency program at that point that the list of interns, and particularly residents with their departments, is incomplete as to department assignments.

General surgery residents started rotating to Austin from St. Joseph Hospital in Houston in 1969, as noted earlier. This arrangement was organized under Dr. Pape's directions and with the help of the other surgeons. Dr. Kenneth Fannin was in that first class as the chief resident in surgery. That program continued under the supervision of the CTMF until the late 1990's.

In 1974 Dr. Clyde Smith was asked to take over management of the surgery program and be its first director. A 1969 graduate of St. Louis Medical School he did his internship in Galveston followed by general surgery at Michael Reese in Chicago. He completed his training in Galveston. His mother and brother lived in Austin, so he decided to come here and work in the emergency room. In his training in general surgery, he was involved in the care of a number of patients in critical care. With his interest in general surgery and critical care in the intensive care unit, he was asked by Raleigh Ross and Maurice Hood if he would consider supervising the general surgery training program under the newly formed CTMF. He accepted that responsibility and set up the call rotation, grand rounds, and worked with the other conferences that were already established such as in pathology. The community surgeons had been involved, as always, but he worked hard to get them to actually turn over the surgeries and the majority of the care to the residents to improve their experience. The decision to perform an operation on a patient is a critical element of the patient care. Having the residents actually be involved in that decision-making process of patient care was of great importance. That decision for private patients and elective surgery would have been made in the doctor's office. The "no-preference" (mostly uninsured) patients, who showed up in the ER, were the ones for whom Dr. Smith wanted the residents to have primary responsibility. Drs. Tom Coopwood, Charlie Ross, and Celia and Wil Van Wisse were particularly helpful in that regard. Dr. Raleigh Ross, as the older surgeon in the group, was a great mentor. He had a variety of older techniques that were not in the repertoire of the current surgeons but were quite helpful in certain cases. This was very much a hands-on program for the residents, in some contrast to the experience in more "academic programs."

Dr. Smith had experience using the flexible colonoscope in his training and was able to pass that experience on to the residents. He started doing flexible gastroscopies as well. Brackenridge did not have flexible gastroscope equipment available so he used the colonoscopes, much to the surgical nurse supervisor's distress. Cleaning the colonoscopes for use in the mouth, esophagus, and stomach was basically distasteful but was certainly something that could be done. One of the long-standing problems at Brackenridge with the city budget was the difficulty of purchasing expensive equipment and keeping current with new trends. That issue has remained a problem for years. It is, however, not unique to Brackenridge as it plagues most hospitals from time to time. On one occasion the gastroscope was damaged. The nurse blamed Dr. Smith and took her concerns to the hospital board. During this investigation, the equipment manufacturer noted that the damage had occurred when the scope had been bitten. That ruled out colonoscopy as the cause for the damage and put a little humor into the situation.

The Swan Ganz Catheter, for monitoring heart function in critical care patients, was a technique that Dr. Smith had used in his training. This technique was becoming an integral part of critical care and was introduced to Brackenridge in his patient care. The procedure involves introducing a catheter into a vein, passing it through the right side of the heart and into the pulmonary artery. In this manner one can record pulmonary arterial pressure, wedge pressure (the back flow pressure coming from the left side of the pulmonary system), overall cardiac function, as well as oxygen levels. In caring for patients in the intensive care unit, the residents became proficient with this new and useful tool.

Surgical Grand Rounds turned out to be a challenging conference for the staff, residents and, particularly, Dr. Smith. The surgeons involved regularly were Drs. Tom Kirksey, Maurice Hood, Hap Arnold, Jimmy Calhoon, Bob Tate and the others listed above, in addition to Dr. Bryan Forrester. Dr. Forrester was a surgeon who had come to town in the late 1960's. Dr. Forester had had a practice in Houston and had actually been a mentor in the anatomy laboratory at Baylor College of Medicine in 1961 when I was a student. We, as very ambitious students, actually felt we knew more anatomy than he did, in spite of his mentoring position.

In any conference, including those in Austin, it is sometimes difficult to get the conversation going. Dr. Smith would occasionally call on Dr. Bryan Forrester with a question, if things seemed to be going slowly, because he knew that several of the other doctors did not want Dr. Forrester to have the last word. This would entice them to jump into the discussion quickly and that would get everything going. Some of Dr. Forrester's comments were not the standard treatment approach that the other doctors thought appropriate for teaching the residents. Dr. Hap Arnold was a good teacher and Dr. Smith wanted his comments in the discussion. Dr. Bill Hart was quiet and was notable for taking the residents "under his wing, gently guiding them through a problem and turning their thinking in the right direction," according to Dr. Smith. Dr. Bud Dryden continuing his long time commitment to the program and was a strong teacher.[49]

Dr. Smith remained the director of surgery until the late 1970's. At that point he chose to start including a private practice for non-clinic patients. Dr. Bob Tate, a cardiovascular surgeon on the staff, decided that was inconsistent with the training program directorship and Dr. Smith chose to leave for full time private practice. CTMF hired Dr. Collins, a Vanderbilt University trained surgeon, to handle the program. Unfortunately, he had some chronic kidney failure that limited his time and energy. In his private practice, Dr. Smith joined the practice of Dr. Reighly Ross, Dr. Tom Coopwood and Dr. Charlie Ross. The education committee of the CTMF asked Dr. Smith if he would return to the management of the surgical service as part of his work with the residents in his private practice. Dr. Collins needed help, so Dr. Smith was part time surgical director between 1980 and [82] as Dr. Collins became progressively less involved with the program and finally left.

The annals of history get foggy with some of the stories that are related by the residents of various services. This story was passed down to a number of residents. A surgical case was discussed on rounds one day and there was concern that proper skin care would be provided in a patient, specifically to the sacral area and tailbone. That is a common area of breakdown when patients are bedfast. In this case the chief resident requested that a "donut" be obtained for the patient to protect the skin. He, of course, meant a rubber round donut to relieve pressure on the sacrum. The intern took it much more literally and got a real donut for the purpose. It is not recorded whether this was glazed or one with icing, but the chief resident was not amused. I think the intern would have been well served to offer up in response long-standing medical treatment where sugar is used in wounds to accelerate granulation tissue and decrease the bacterial load. It is not recorded whether this excuse was used.

In 1982, Dr. David H. Harshaw, Jr. became the medical director of the surgical teaching service. He was a native of Pennsylvania and a 1957 Graduate of the University of Pennsylvania. He competed his surgical training in Philadelphia and joined a practice there. He was drafted in 1966 and soon found himself in Viet Nam. He was assigned to the 93rd evacuation hospital were he would cross paths the Dr. Don Patrick and Dr. Edwin Buster, two neurosurgeons he would later see in Austin. He was involved in setting up this relatively new military hospital in Viet Nam, organizing meetings and research projects, as well as a journal club and an interesting case conference daily. On returning to civilian life he joined the trauma service at Down State King's County Hospital. He later was part of the oncology service. That service needed some expertise in head and neck surgery so Dave went as a fellow to M.D. Anderson Hospital in Houston from 1969 to 1970. By 1975 there were some problems in the Down State department, so he joined a friend in practice in New Mexico. That worked well for his wife, a physicist, who took a job at Los Alamos. The original partner rejoined the military and in 1982 the opening in Central Texas Medical Foundation became available. He was recruited in part by Dr. Smith and so another move was in order. Dr. Harshaw had a broad range of training and experience and was the outstanding applicant for the job.

On coming to Austin, he found the program here somewhat less organized than he anticipated. There had been significant progress over the previous ten years, but the lack of continuity in management experience did show. Dr. Clyde Smith was busy with a private practice and was only part time with the training program and Dr. Collins had left. The department consisted of one secretary, four residents rotating up from St. Joseph Hospital in Houston, and four transitional interns in Family Practice and Internal medicine. Dr. Harshaw started early building a good relationship with St. Joseph and, as a result, getting good residents. There were second, third, fourth year residents plus the chief resident. They rotated up for four months at a time, and, since they came back each year, the staff got to know then and their strengths and weaknesses. The mortality and morbidity, trauma and Saturday conferences were strengthened. The continuing support of the community general surgeons remained a strong element of the program. Again Drs. Coopwood, Charlie Ross, Vasquez, Hart, Van Weises, Church and Bridges were very active. Dr. Harshaw did vascular surgery but was also doing much of the pediatric surgery. Dr. Abe Bessserman, trained in pediatric surgery, came to Austin and Dr. Hart began doing pediatric surgery. Dr. Harshaw was glad to have them involved. Eventually, Dr. Schlecter, also a pediatric surgeon joined the community and performed much of the pediatric general surgery.

In 1992, a Level II trauma accreditation was achieved. Attaining that level required a detailed accounting of trauma cases, surgeries, research, neurosurgery coverage, Advanced Certified Live Support (ACLS) certification of the surgeons, and a burn unit. The burn unit was available in San Antonio, at Brook Army Hospital. Dr. Jose Bravo, a partner of surgeon Dr. Hector Morales became director of the trauma service. He was quite detail oriented and made sure all of the complex practice requirements were accomplished and recorded. Eventually a Level I accreditation was achieved.

Dr. Hector Morales came to Austin as a general surgeon and planned to join a practice in South Austin. That association did not work as he had hoped and a transition from that arrangement occurred. He became active at Brackenridge and started ER call as a community general surgeon in 1977. He had done his general surgery residency, followed by a vascular surgery fellowship at Henry Ford Hospital in Detroit. He remained active at Brackenridge and was asked by Dr. Don Spencer to become a member of the CTMF board. In 1990 he was elected president of the CTMF board and remained in that position for 8 years. The budget for the training program, with all the departments went from about $2,000,000 to the range of $7-8,000,000 during his tenure. He became centrally involved in discussions with Seton and its potential for taking over the management of the hospital and training program.[50]

The work load at Brackenridge for community doctors, covering the emergencies in the emergency room, doing surgeries when necessary and following those patients in the hospital had become quite time consuming. In some cases it interfered with seeing patients in a private practice. Spending the night in the ER or in the operating room made work the next day difficult. Some doctors dropped off the list of those willing to covering the ER. As an incentive to continue call, some of the services began to pay the doctors for the night's work. The practice had been initiated by the neurosurgeons in the late 1980's, followed shortly by general surgery, orthopedics, and other services. With the pay for night call on general surgery, came the requirement that the general surgeons would have to stay overnight in the hospital to cover the service. Eventually, it was found to be necessary to have a list of back up surgeons available to cover when things got really busy. With over one hundred and ten emergency room calls per month, almost four per day, many involving serious injuries and subsequent surgery, the workload was extreme. Sometimes the back up doctor had to come in and help with the chaos. This level of intensity was not uncommon in busy emergency rooms across the country.[51]

As the leadership of the various services evolved, the next candidate for the surgery service, Dr. Ben Coopwood, son of surgeon, Dr. Thomas Coopwood, graduated from the University of Texas at Houston in 1990. He completed his surgical residency at Baylor in Houston and moved to Austin with his family in 1995. He joined the surgical practice of Drs. Tom Coopwood, Charlie Ross and Clyde Smith. After a year, as things were changing in private practice he looked at other possibilities in Austin but also in Houston. His wife did not want to move back to Houston. He had been active at Brackenridge and in discussion with Dr. Harshaw some money was found to provide a position as director for the Transitional Internship section. Dr. Coopwood would continue to be involved with the surgical service but would also be responsible for the rotation assignments, service assignments, teaching conferences and recruiting for each year.

In 1995, the Seton Hospital System took over the administration of Brackenridge under contract with the City. That change was so abrupt that when Earl Matthews, (Medical Director of all the programs), took the budget to the City, the budget office redirected him to Seton saying that Seton had the money from the City to cover the training program. It appears that there may have been a little sleight of hand on the part of the City, since the Travis County Medical Society was still managing the training program and received some of that training money from the City. The budget that Dr. Matthews took to Seton was around $7 million. They said they had $5 million. The arrangement was finally settled for the time being. The budgeting process, however, created some friction between Seton and Dr. Matthews, who had been director for twenty years.

Dr. Matthews chose that time to make a major change in his work for good or bad. He chose to leave the program and to pursue an infections disease practice in Corpus Christi. Dr. Jose Brave, who had been the lead person in obtaining a level II emergency room rating, was also let go by Seton. On the other hand, the new management was helpful to the surgery department because at least some more money became available for such equipment as laparoscopes and endoscopes. Some of the surgical equipment had been borrowed from other facilities in the past. That may sound strange, but a great deal of equipment was borrowed back and forth for years, particularly between St. David's and Brackenridge in surgery, orthopedics and gynecology.

Within the first few years of Seton management, several changes followed. Much of it had to do with budgeting. Around 2000 they considered eliminating more faculty positions, including the position of Transitional Intern director, Ben Coopwood's job. At that time Dr. Harshaw was considering reducing his activities. Ultimately, Ben moved into more of the management responsibilities of the surgery department and eventually became the chief while Dr. Harshaw assumed the Transitional Intern program as a part time position. The surgery residents from St. Joseph continued to rotate to Austin during their third, fourth and chief resident years. Austin was responsible for the salaries of the residents since we benefited from their medical services and patient care. That system evolved such that the first and second year residents were coming to Austin by 2006.

In the early 2000's, a strange sequence of events in Houston affected the program in Austin. Baylor College of Medicine decided that, to be a top rated institution, it needed to own an outpatient clinic and a hospital. Since 1944 their main teaching hospital had been Methodist Hospital. In addition, St. Luke's Hospital, Texas Children's Hospital, Jefferson Davis, Herman Memorial, and later Ben Taub hospitals had joined as teaching facilities over the years. The desire of Baylor to have its own facilities created a major conflict with Methodist that eventually resulted in a break up of their long-standing relationship. Baylor had the "ownership" of the residency programs at Methodist and Baylor elected to withdraw the residents from Methodist. This, of course, created a vacuum in coverage and teaching at Methodist. At about the same time, St. Joseph Hospital, the downtown Houston hospital from which the surgery residents rotated to Austin, was having some difficulty maintaining all of its services and considered closing. For whatever reason, Methodist Hospital managed to take over the accredited surgical residency training positions from St. Joseph by 2004. The Austin program tried to work out a rotation for the residual St. Joseph residents to allow for a phased coverage arrangement as the residents were withdrawn from Austin. They were unable to develop as satisfactory agreement and, thus, all of the residents were withdrawn from Austin. That meant that for the years 2006 to 2008, there were no residents at St. Joseph or Methodist to be sent to Austin. This left the general surgery staff, including Dr. Harshaw, Dr. Ben Coopwood, and the "Space Cowboys," to cover the entire surgery service. "Space Cowboys" was a term applied by the residents, derived from a movie about old astronauts hired to dismantle old satellites. This group included Dr. Tom Coopwood, Dr. Jose Bravo and Dr. Tom Kirksey, all of whom came out of retirement to covered the entire trauma and general surgery service, including ER and outpatient clinics, for almost two years between 2006 and 2008. Their primary responsibility was to make sure the clinics were covered and to make hard medical decisions with the transitional interns and students. This was an extremely heavy workload for these loyal doctors.

Other issues, some outside of Austin, would continue to affect the program here. Discussions in Galveston involved the possibility of more affiliation between that institution and the training programs in Austin. Ultimately, it would be helpful to both programs to have an arrangement whereby Austin could benefit from the UTMB experience and UTMB could utilize the patient population in Austin for students and residents.

The rotation of UTMB residents in surgery continued through 2008. At that time another event in history would interrupt the arrangement between UT Medical Branch and the Austin training program. In the fall of 2008, Hurricane Ike, the most expensive tropical storm in U. S. history, struck the Texas coast near Galveston and wrought havoc on the city, including the medical school. Many of the buildings were flooded, research facilities were damaged and John Sealy hospital was closed for a year. The cost of damage to the medical complex was estimated at $1 Billion. This resulted in huge financial concerns and the layoff of nearly 3,000 employees. There was even discussion by the University of Texas Board of Regents of moving the school off the island. That idea was not implemented but it took six years to rebuild the campus. Medical students were farmed out mostly to Baylor in Houston. Continuing with the joint program with Austin was considered no longer feasible because of the difficulty of financing the designated institutional officer, supporting the residents, and contributing to the Austin faculty. There had been quite a lot of discussion with UTMB about dissolving the relationship months before the hurricane arrived so it was not entirely the weather that resulted in the dissolution of the relationship. There was great concern about cost and there was concern by the Galveston faculty about the relationship with Austin. They were particularly worried about the continued pressure to move the medical school, perhaps to Austin, a proposition for which they were not supportive.

In 2009 the overall coordination of the various training programs in Austin was transferred to University of Texas Southwestern Medical School in Dallas. They could provide help with accreditation and other administrative functions. In the same year, as a result of the disruption of the management work by UTMB and the end of coordinating programs in Galveston and Houston, the surgery section decided to go an independent route and start a surgical program of its own. After significant work, they achieved accreditation and elected to apply to the resident matching program for first year residents only. In that way they could add a new class each year, develop their own residents from the start, and not fill the second, third and fourth year slots with residents transferred in from other programs. Thus, in 2014, the first full class of general surgery residents completed their four-year program in Austin.[51,52]

In January of 2015, Dr. Ben Coopwood was made Assistant Professor and named Vice-Chair of the Department of Surgery for UT Austin Dell Medical School as it became operational. There are currently 10 faculty members on the surgery department staff with a trauma section, a surgical critical care unit, a breast care center, a vascular surgery section, and the trauma center of Brackenridge.

Obstetrics and Gynecology

Dr. Georgia Leggett (noted earlier in this text) maintained a strong connection with Dr. Willard Cook, the chairman of the obstetrics and gynecology department at UTMB where she attended medical school. Dr. Cook guided and encouraged her in her postgraduate training in Houston, Philadelphia, New Jersey and New York. When she moved to Austin they discussed the possibility of some type of training program to be developed at Brackenridge beyond the internship program. She, along with Dr. F. K. Blewett, chairman of the obstetrics section at Brackenridge, set up a program in which UTMB residents would come to Austin for part of their training. Dr. Frank Lee was the first resident in ob./gyn. to spend time at Brackenridge.

In 1955 four student externs came to Austin and along with a resident by the name of Dr. Joseph Durso. In the 1956-57 year there were three residents and the program grew from that point. In the mid 1960's, with the establishment of a more formal training program under Dr. Pape, these residents were included under that umbrella. Drs. Legett, McCulley, Blewett, Weaver and Harrod were trained obstetrician/gynecologists and they were supported by at least seven general practitioners who included obstetrics in their practice. They all supervised the residents with deliveries and the obstetricians helped in the surgeries. Many of these doctors remained active in the program for many years.[18]

Dr. Fred Hansen arrived in Austin in 1964 to start his OB/Gyn. practice. As a new doctor at Brackenridge, the primary place to start your practice, he joined the staff. Essentially all departments had an understanding that the staff doctors would cover call in the emergency room on a rotating basis, see patients in the public clinics, and support the residents in their activities. This was particularly true for the new doctors in town. The only exception to this practice was the urology service where the new doctor would cover Brackenridge until another new urologist came to town. That could be several years. Dr. Hansen continued at Brackenridge for 8-10 years and then turned his duties over to the younger doctors arriving in town.[53]

With the formation in 1972 of the Central Texas Medical Foundation the next step in formalizing the ob./gyn. training program was taken. Dr. Tad Davis, a local practicing physician, was hired to run the residency training. He would be responsible for developing a curriculum, a rotation schedule, the clinic coverage, and the involvement of the many doctors from the community who contributed to direct service and training. There were assignments to the clinic for both residents and supervising doctors and there was a night call schedule for both. Dr. Davis not only was busy with his private practice but he was also an avid flyer. Some of the residents indicated that he was frequently out flying and thus was not always present in the hospital when they thought they needed help on some cases. As noted earlier, under the discussion of Dr. Legett's involvement in the 1950's and 1960's, the staff did not cover all routine deliveries but would be involve in complicated deliveries and cesarean sections, and come to the hospital for surgeries.

The residents at that time continued to be from the UTMB program. Interestingly, in the list of house staff there are lists of flexible interns and family practice, internal medicine and surgery residents, but no listing of the ob./gyn. residents. I assume that since the program was run by UTMB, Brackenridge did not keep track of that program in the same manner. Generally, there were three or four residents at a time considering the four-year program.

In 1975, Dr. Clyde Dorr was hired as acting director and then advanced to full time director. He, along with Dr. Mark Reidel, ran the program while the community doctors maintained a very active part in patient care and resident supervision. Dr. Dorr was a sharp dresser. He was always seen in a coat and tie and usually a hat. He remained as director through the tenure of the UTMB program and then remained as an active participant in the part time faculty as he developed a private practice, mostly at St. David's. Eventually he was recruited to Houston and finally moved to Gainesville Florida to a faculty position.

Dr. Terry Kuhlmann arrived in Austin in 1977 to set up practice in ob./gyn. He joined the staff at Brackenridge and joined the call schedule to cover the ER, see patients in surgery, rotate with the residents, come in for back up of residents in the delivery room and assist with surgeries as necessary. He and his partners Drs. Chris Wilson, Bruno Ybarra, and John Baker were among the community doctors that covered these responsibilities.[54]

In 1977, Dr. Eldrid Kaplan joined the ob./gyn. department at the University of Texas at Houston Medical School. He had graduated from the University of Cape Town Medical School, South Africa in 1967. He completed his residency there, followed by two years in a teaching position. As did many recent graduates in South Africa, he went to England and worked as a junior registrar in the national health system. He had the unique experience of a period in Israel. He then applied for a teaching job at the University of Texas, Houston, Obstetrics and Gynecology department at the suggestion of Dr. Paul Weinberg who was then the director at UT San Antonio. U. T. Houston held the job for him for a year, as he navigated the United States immigration system. Shortly after his arrival in Houston, there was discussion of UTMB withdrawing from the Austin program. In 1979, UTMB did, in fact, withdraw their OB/Gyn. residents from Austin and the University of Texas, Houston, started rotating their residents here. Since, according to Dr. Kaplan, one of the decision makers on the board of regents was particularly indecisive, UT Houston physically took over the program and began rotating residents here several months before the decision came from the regents. The Houston program sought a director for Austin, and after a weekend visit to Austin, Dr. Kaplan eagerly took the position.[55]

It was anticipated that taking over the program in Austin would lead to a significant number of operational complications, particularly because the obstetrics protocols being used at UT Houston might be different from those in Austin. Protocols in labor and delivery or standards of care included activities such as when to artificially induce labor, when to do C-sections, what anesthesia would be used, and other practices that may vary from community to community. The faculty in Houston specifically chose Dr. Allen Stringer, the chief resident at the time, to lead the way as the first resident in Austin. He was very well versed in the practice and had a strong personality; he would not be intimidated by push-back from nursing or consulting hospital staff doctors in Austin. It is not uncommon for the mature nursing staff in obstetrics to have little question about how things are to be done. In many cases they question the need for doctors in the obstetrical process. They could be quite dogmatic about how things were to be done. Dr. Stringer apparently managed very well in this potential mine field. Following Dr. Stringer, Dr. Jerald Mankovsky rotated here to become the chief resident. He was reluctant to come but firmly encouraged to come to Austin for a reason similar to Dr. Stringer's. He remembers the time here as being extremely busy. He said that they would frequently start surgeries at 7:30 in the morning and would not finish until 8:00 in the evening. He found it to be great experience with good support from the staff. He had graduated from Texas Tech Medical School in 1976 and started his residency in St. Louis at the Barnes and Jewish hospital. He did not find that program to his satisfaction and transferred to the Houston program. The University of Texas at Houston was only eight years old at the time.[56]

Dr. Kaplan found the medical community very supportive of the program. As they had done in the past, they rotated coverage of the emergency room, covered the clinics with the residents, and frequently came in to cover surgeries and complicated deliveries with the residents.

A challenge in this community was the lack of regularly available epidural anesthesia services. Epidural anesthesia for obstetrics was not taught as the norm in anesthesia residencies across the country. That service was, however, available in Houston. Epidural anesthesia required an anesthesiologist to be present in the hospital for the duration of the procedure and this was much more costly and time intensive for all. It was, however, becoming considered a safer alternative to other forms of anesthesia in obstetrics. With time it became the standard for vaginal deliveries, cesarean sections, and other lower abdominal procedures. There was a group of anesthesiologists who had faithfully provided services at Brackenridge for years, including Drs. Johnson, Umstad, and Yeakel. They chose to limit their hours and to not provide routine epidural services at Brackenridge. In 1974 Drs. Dennis Boyer, Doughty, and Richard Shoberg came to town as a new group. Dr. Boyer and Dr. Doughty had had special training with the military in providing anesthesia for acute trauma and they wanted to practice at Brackenridge. On arrival in Austin, they chose to provide epidural anesthesia for obstetrics at Seton and at Brackenridge. This provided them an edge to compete in the anesthesia market of Austin. Over the next six to eight years they increased their presence in both Seton and Brackenridge and influenced the entire anesthesia community to provide those services. As a consequence, by the late 1970's and early 1980's, as Dr. Kaplan was establishing the training service for Houston residents, epidural anesthesia became more available, making obstetrical services more comfortable for all, especially the laboring mothers. Drs. Johnson, Lassiter and Yeakel had practiced at St. David's as well as Brackenridge. In the late 1970's they chose to move their entire practice from Brackenridge to St. David's rather that provide epidurals to obstetrics. However, it was not that many years until epidural anesthesia became more popular throughout the community so that Drs. Johnson, Lassiter and Yeakel's and new partners at St. David's were providing that procedure routinely. Times change and the community of medicine changes with it.[57]

Dr. Mankovsky decided to move to Austin in 1980 when he finished in Houston. He started a solo practice but immediately joined the staff at Brackenridge and became involved with the teaching program. He was appointed to be a clinical assistant professor of UT Houston and then promoted to associate professor. He spent two full days per week with the residents in clinics, in surgery, and as back up in labor and delivery. He also developed a series of lectures for the residents and included the Family Practice residents and students rotating up from the Houston medical school. There were not many formal lectures prior to this effort by Dr. Mankovsky. As part of the ob./gyn. department, he took emergency room call in rotation with the rest of the department. Heavily involved in the activities of the department were Drs. Joseph DesRosiers, Nobel Doss, Brad Price, Jo Quander, Eric Upton, and Al Gross plus the others in Dr. Kuhlmann's group. In the early 1980's the department set a policy that to be on staff at Brackenridge one had to cover the emergency room for, not only back up of the residents, but all Obstetrics and gynecology in the emergency room. This was done because the patient load continued to climb and many hands were needed. This, on the other hand, required the private physicians to cover a large number of gynecological problems that were beyond the scope of the time commitment that they were willing endure. This resulted in resignation of some of the community doctors from the department.

Dr. Kaplan remained department head for about two years, followed by five or more years as part time faculty as he transferred his energies into his own private practice. Dr. Mankovsky became the acting director and the search was on for a new director. Dr. Allen Stringer, the former resident, was hired for a short time to be the director. He helped with the program until a new director was hired. Dr. Stringer eventually became head of the gynocological oncology services for the state-wide Texas Oncology group. The new head of the ob./gyn. service was Dr. Kavoussi, who was originally from Iran. He was hired as director and remained with the program for 3-4 years. He was considered not a strong director and had somewhat limited surgical skill.[56]

Dr. Eric Upton graduated from Baylor College of Medicine in 1977. He completed his OB/Gyn. training at Baylor as well. He came to Austin in 1981 and joined the staff at Brackenridge. He began the routine service of night call in the emergency room, saw patients in the clinics on a rotating basis and was part of the volunteer staff assisting the residents. When he admitted some of his own private patients to the hospital, the residents would frequently scrub in on his surgeries. In addition, he would help by scrubbing in on their C-sections. After four to five years, he was asked to become part of the paid UT Houston part time faculty as he was spending a full day a week in the clinic in addition to the surgeries. He remained on the faculty until 1989. It was at that time that the residents from Houston were withdrawn from Austin.

Dr. Upton reduced his involvement but continued to provide services. At present he works within the County Health Department to provide many of the services that are not available at Seton. He helps with counseling patients and providing birth control prescriptions and devices. With new technology he is able to insert devises to block the fallopian tube endoscopically, as an office procedure, in additions to standard intrauterine devises (IUDs) also as an outpatient. He retains a position of the faculty, now with the new University of Texas Dell Medical School.[58]

In 1990, the Lyndon B. Johnson Hospital in Houston opened in affiliation with the UT Medical School. This new hospital would create a significant increase in the workload for doctors in the various residency programs. Dr. Robert Creasy was the director in obstetrics in Houston and a nationally known physician. He initially stated that they would keep their residents in Austin but found that they were going to be stretched too thin to cover both Houston and Austin. Therefore their residents were withdrawn from rotations in Austin. As a consequence, an arrangement was made with the St. Joseph program in Houston to rotate their residents here. Dr. Joe Lucci was the program director at St. Joseph. This was the same program that had rotated general surgery residents to Austin since 1969. Dr. Upton was asked to be the director of the department and was also asked to put together a group of qualified doctors to assist with mentoring the residents. This requirement illustrates an evolution in committed community doctors in the various services involved with the teaching responsibilities. The group that agreed to help with the residents included Drs. Brian Manks, Paul Locus, Robin Braun, Mary Gasal, and Jodi Moore. There were three residents for each year. Following Dr. Upton, Dr. Paul Locus became the director two to three years.

In the mid 1990's things became quite complicated with the training programs and the hospital in general. Mr. Dandridge was the hospital administrator at the time. There had developed an assortment of payment arrangements with the various training sections and variable and changing payment schedules for private doctors who covered emergency room call and clinic responsibilities. A question arose regarding these payment schedules and how many rules were being bent to accommodate the personalities and demands of the various interests. The administrator seemed to handle these arrangements by keeping the pay schedules secret to prevent interdepartmental competition. Managing these complications along with the leadership responsibilities of the program itself became quite burdensome. As a consequence, a full time head of the department was felt to be the logical next step.

Dr. Charles E. L Brown grew up in Dallas and then attended undergraduate and medical school at Tulane, graduating in 1980. Having grown up with a very handy father and working as a scrub technician at Charity hospital in New Orleans, he chose the surgical field of Obstetrics and Gynecology. His residency was at UTMB in Galveston. Fellowships were not common at the time but one of his mentors encouraged him, so he went on to Parkland in Maternal-Fetal Medicine (MFM), the care of complicated pregnancies. He stayed on the faculty in Dallas. When his sister, a single mother, developed melanoma, she asked Dr. Brown to consider supporting her son through college. Dr. Brown decided that private practice would make that more practical financially, so he chose a practice in Austin with Dr. Bryan Darby and, later, Dr. Robert Patterson, both specializing in maternal-fetal medicine. After Dr. Brown moved to Austin in 1994, in addition to the private practice, Seton requested that he work for them part time as a medical director involving MFM. That involved about 10-15 % of his workload. He was about to enter the convoluted administration of Seton, Brackenridge, the City, community doctors at Brackenridge, the medical staff and the residency program involving St Joseph doctors in training.

At a staff meeting at Seton in 1994, Mr. Charles Barnett, CEO of Seton, announced that a contract with the City to take over management of Brackenridge was eminent.

By 1998. Seton acquired the oversight of the training programs at Brackenridge and by 1999 Dr. Brown was working about 50% of his time with Seton, Seton Northwest, and Brackenridge; and 50% with his private practice. His private practice allowed him to get to know many OB and primary care doctors all over central Texas, as he and his practice were the referral center for complicated pregnancies. As part of his Seton responsibilities he was made chairman of the Quality Care Council, that would have strong control of many of the department policies.

With the Seton take-over of obstetrical services, there were more complications to encounter. Seton, as a Catholic institution, could not provide contraception, sterilization or pregnancy termination services. Their solution was to create a "hospital within a hospital" concept that would separate the fifth floor of the hospital as a completely separate institution from Brackenridge. This would mean that the fifth floor would be isolated as a separate hospital, involving building a separate elevator and even transporting surgical instruments back and forth to Houston, where they could be sterilized outside of Brackenridge main facilities. Seton relinquished the management of the fifth floor back to the City. The City never actually managed that program since this arrangement development coincided with UTMB management of the training programs in the early 2000's. There were long meetings to work out compromises for certain services, such as emergency resuscitation code responses between Brackenridge main hospital and this Women's hospital.[58,59] They initially managed post partum tubal ligations by outsourcing these services, mostly to St. David's. That was a problem as it delayed the tubal surgery for six weeks rather than provide an easier surgery at the time of the delivery. All provisions for birth control had to be handled outside the hospital. With a large indigent population who had no other source of these women's services, the problems were daunting. In 1999, the council of Catholic Bishops concluded that this program by Seton to deal with the reproductive services could not continue. Further modifications would be necessary.

At this point the residents from St. Joseph were coming to Austin for four months at a time. In addition, Dr. Earl Matthews, under his tenure, had started a fellowship program for family practice residents to provide them with a year of training in obstetrics. This provided needed obstetrical training and allowed some of them to perform C-sections in the practices they would eventually establish. A number of students rotated up from UTMB in Galveston for their clerkships in obstetrics. Dr. Mark Peters was hired to deal with the obstetrics programs as it was rather complicated with all of the different trainees from different programs.

By 2001-2, Dr. Brown was spending 50-60 % of his time with the program. In addition to the residents, fellows and students, the high volume of deliveries allowed the department to establish relationships with family medicine residency programs in Wyoming, Albuquerque, New Mexico, Corpus Christi, and San Antonio for their obstetrics rotations through the Brackenridge program.

In the ever-changing environment of dictums from on high, the Accreditation Council for Graduate Medical Education, (ACGME), the agency formed by the American Medical Association and Medicare/Medicaid in a compromise of control by medicine and federal financing, stated that a functioning training program needed a full time director. So, in 2003, Dr. Brown resigned from his private practice and became the full time director.

St. Joseph's training program was having some financial problems and Methodist Hospital in Houston was losing its residents. Methodist looked to the program at St. Joseph for help. In additions, considering the long-standing relationship in obstetrics from the 1950's, UTMB was exploring the idea of creating an affiliated satellite program in Austin. Dr. Al LeBlanc, the Designated Institutional Official emeritus under Dr. Tom Blackwell the DIO at Galveston, helped draw up the new program in partnership with Dr. Brown and Dr. Jim Lindsey, V.P. at Seton. This program would be a separate and distinct program from the ongoing residency program at Galveston. This new program achieved approval in March of 2004 from the American College of Graduate Medical Education. It was decided, that in order to control the resident applicants more closely, the program would register for applicants for the first year residents/transitional interns matching program for the year 2005. There were plenty of students, family practice fellows and residents from other programs who could manage the patient load. The first four-year graduates completed their training in 2009 and by 2015, 34 residents had completed the new Austin obstetrics and gynecology program.

Dr. Brown has continued to be head of the Austin program and is responsible for the care and handling of the students from Galveston. They required nurturing, so Dr. Ted Held was hired to assist with that responsibility. Dr. Brown was also made a vice dean at UTMB so that he could run the Quality Improvement meetings at Brackenridge. There was also a complicated payment arrangement between Seton and Galveston to pay for the residents and staff in Austin. This varied and changeable program was the result of having residents from other programs over the years. This was in marked contrast to the relative stability of the pediatric and internal medicine programs that were independent Austin programs from the start of CTMF.[59] Developing an independent training program in ob./gyn. starting in 2005 clearly simplified the management by eliminating the variations involved in residents rotating from other communities.

In 2008 hurricane Ike struck Galveston and destroyed much of the medical school. That, among other factors, drastically changed the relationship with Austin and UTMB withdrew from Austin programs. Ultimately, all of the sections in Austin came under the administrative assistance of the University of Texas Southwestern in Dallas, where a new Designated Institutional Official would be available. That responsibility would eventually be transferred to the Dell Medical School.

After Galveston withdrew from the Austin program and the University of Texas Southwestern administration became the administrator, the fifth floor "hospital within a hospital" facility that allowed Seton to manage the obstetrics program was eventually closed. Most of the obstetrics functions were transferred to St. David's hospital, where a great deal of Medicaid obstetrics had been handled for some time. Other portions of that service have been gradually transferred to the Seton main hospital except for cases in which there is anticipation of post partum tubal ligation services. It is anticipated that there will be no labor and delivery service at the new UT Dell Medical School so the residents will be busy traveling. They will need to go the Dell Children's Hospital for some newborns, Brackenridge for some gynecological services and Seton for deliveries and other newborn services such as circumcision.[59]

Other contributors to the ob./gyn. department have been Dr. Thomas Vaughn and his partners at the Texas Fertility Center. Three areas of training, in addition to the basic services for Ob/Gyn., need to be part of the modern training program for residents. These include infertility, maternal fetal medicine and oncology. Dr. Charles Brown is a maternal fetal medicine specialist providing those specialized services and training in cases of pregnancies complicated by issues such as diabetes mellitus, hypertension, and other issues that can be a threat to the mother or child. He is, therefore, the primary source for training in that area. Dr. Ellen B. Smith, Dr. Mark A Corzier, and other doctors at Texas Oncology have provided the experience and training for the residents in cancer treatment. Dr. Vaughn and his associated have been the resource for training in infertility. Dr. Vaughn did his medical school training and his residency at UTMB, completing that program in 1978. He spent a year on the faculty there, and then followed with a two-year fellowship in infertility/reproductive endocrinology at Duke University. He then moved to Austin, and in 1983, with the help of St. David's hospital, opened one of the first in vitro fertilization (IVF) programs in the country. That service expanded and, again with the partnership with St. David's hospital, built a surgical facility on north Mopac in 2006. As the services are so specialized and require special equipment, the residents come to their offices for this subspecialty training rather than staying at Brackenridge. In that training period they gain experience in oocyte retrieval, gamete intrafallopian transfers (GIFT), and cryopreservation (freezing) of embryos. They have added donor oocytes, donor sperm, gestational carriers and oocyte cryopreservation services to patient care as these new techniques have become part of Obstetrics practice and a necessary part of the training of the residents. Dr. Vaughn and others go to Brackenridge to provide didactic lectures for the residents as well. There was a time when UTMB residents came to Austin for fellowship training in infertility but that stopped in 2008 with the disruption of many programs with UTMB.[60]

In January of 2015, Dr. Amy Young, formerly of the LSU Medial School, was appointed to the chairmanship of the ob./gyn. department, under the UT Dell Medical School.

As noted earlier, by 2015 there were thirty-four residents who had complete the full four-year residency. They had achieved a 100% passing rate for the obstetrics/gynecology boards and seven had been accepted to fellowship programs. This seems a remarkable record for a community-based training program and attests to the outstanding local expertise.[59]

Family Medicine

For generations, most medical doctors practiced as General Practitioners. They saw the medical problems in both adults and children; treated general surgery patients and did the surgeries; delivered babies; set fractures; and offered all of the services available in medicine. As time passed, more and more doctors studied the specialties of ear, nose and throat surgery, general surgery, obstetrics and gynecology, pediatrics, orthopedics, etc. General practitioners began to restrict their practices and, in some hospitals, their privileges would be restricted from some areas of specialized services unless they had extra training. The area of general practice evolved into family practice that includes obstetrics. That would be essential, especially in rural areas. family practice was established as a specialty, recognized by the American Board of Medical Specialties, in 1969.[61]

As the Central Texas Medical Foundation was being formed, Drs. Ruth Bain, John Kelly, V. C. Smart, Joe Reneau, and others decided that the community needed to include Family Practice as one of the programs at Brackenridge. After all, the whole point of this community education effort was to provide a full array of doctors to serve the community. This would be a natural extension of the general internship that had been present for forty years.

The pediatric program started in 1972 and by 1974 the family practice program was beginning. 1975 was approaching as the last year that independent rotating internships would be sanctioned by the American Counsel of Graduate Medical Education (ECGME). Dr. Constance Hanna and Dr. Hardy Morgan were in the internship class of 1973-74 and were offered the opportunity to join the new Family Practice program as second year residents, since they has just completed their internship year. Under the directorship of Dr. John Kelly, they accepted and became the first two second-year residents in the program for 1974-75. Therefore, the original director was Dr. John Kelly, a general practitioner in Austin who served for a short period to get the program started. He was followed by Dr. Paul Schedler. Dr. Ruth Bain indicates in her biography that she was a clinical director in the 1974-76 years. Part of that time she was associate director. She also offered her office in the Medical Arts Square as a first location for the outpatient clinic.[62]

Dr. John Smolik graduated from Galveston in 1974 and had applied for a rotating internship at Brackenridge. By the time that he arrived, the internship was integrated into the Family Practice residency and he was assigned as a first year resident or transitional intern. He, along with Drs. Terry Wiggins, Ira Bell, Sidney Robins, and Douglas Wohlfahrt, became the first first-year residents in the program. John had spent about nine of his twelve-month senior year in medical school doing externships in Austin. He had such a good experience that he applied to the program here. He found the program of night call much more than he liked. No matter what rotation he was on, there was still a requirement that he be on call for obstetrics every third night. That he found rather exhausting, although he did acquire a lot of experience delivering babies. As a result, he left the program after his first year and became a full time doctor in the emergency room.

He planned to apply to a psychiatry residency but was redirected by another experience. He became aware of a new clinic, a Minor Emergency Room (Minor ER) on Anderson Lane in north Austin run by Dr. Dennis Ela. After visiting with Dr. Ela and learning about the business, he decided to join Dr. Ela and they opened a second Minor ER in south Austin. This was a first for Austin, and, as there was only one ER in town (at Brackenridge) and general practitioner's and pediatrician's offices were very busy, the minor ERs became very popular and busy. As Dr. Smolick noted, "we became the bad guys in town as we were felt to be stealing patients from the general practitioner's offices." Ah, the problems with "newness." They filled a real need in the community and became incubators for a number of future minor emergency rooms in the city.[63]

Drs. Hanna and Morgan were the first to complete their programs in 1976, and Drs. Ira Bell, Terry Wiggins, Douglas Wolfahrt and Lynn

Warthan all completed their training in 1977. Drs. Hanna, Wohlfahrt, and Warthan all spent a month in our clinic, the Austin Bone and Joint clinic, for their orthopedic experience.[63,64,65] By that time Dr. Schedler had completed his stint as director and he was followed by Dr. Bain as acting director from 1976-77. She remained as associate director when Dr. Glen Johnson became the first non-Austinite hired by CTMF for the directorship. Dr. Johnson was a relatively recent graduate of the Howard University Family Practice Program. When he moved to Austin to practice he was asked by Dr. Earl Matthews to take on the responsibility of running the program. Dr. Mathis Blackstock was quoted as making quite a nice comment about Dr. Johnson. He said that he noted a great deal of respect by Dr. Johnson for the residents. That was in quite a contrast to the way residents were treated in Dr. Blackstock's days of training. In former times it was surprisingly common for residents to be treated as real underlings or worker bees while in training programs. Dr. Johnson was "respectful, thoughtful and considerate." "He just seemed to have a knack for keeping a lid on situations that could have become tense." Dr. Blackstock resolved to incorporate that respect for residents in his own approach. It is evident that he was successful in that effort, as noted in the esteem the residents had for Dr. Blackstock.[66]

The next year, 1978, the staff thought that it would be helpful for the program to move their outpatient clinic facilities away from Dr. Bain's office to a location more accessible for patients. The office of Dr. Bain was becoming limiting because of space. Thus a location was found on E. 49 ½ and I-35. It was a one level building, in the northeast section of the city, with lots of street level parking. So, in addition to the hospital inpatients who required office follow -up after discharge, the residents saw outpatients at this new Family Medicine clinic as well as the Rosewood Zaragosa clinic in east Austin.

Drs. Bain, Blackstock, Kelly, Johnson and others in the family practice section continued to use the outpatient clinic but began to consider the possibilities of a building that would be owned by CTMF and would be specifically designed for use as a clinic. CTMF, Earl Matthews, and the other services were not included in this planning phase. Mr. Marshall Cothran was hired in 1990 by Mr. Tom Young, the CEO of the Travis County Medical Society, to be an assistant administrator, with specific duties to include management of the teaching program. With growth, the teaching program had become much more complex, including approximately 50 employees in administration in addition to the teaching staff and residents in the various programs. Mr. Cothran was to work with Earl Matthews, the current Director of Medical Education. In retrospect, Mr. Cothran felt that his appearance on the Austin scene was probably difficult for Dr. Matthews, who had been managing the training program by himself for fifteen years and reporting directly to the CTMF board. That situation resolved itself with time. At the time Mr. Cothran was hired, the design of the new clinic building was nearly completed and a name, The Blackstock Family Health Care Clinic, had been chosen. It appeared to Mr. Cothran that there was a certain tension in the community between the CTMF board and the Family Medicine doctors, as there had been a lack of communication about the project. In the years between the 1950s and1960s, the medical community had evolved significantly. In the 1950s the predominant physician practices were general practice. Progressively, in the 1970s and beyond, the predominant growth in physicians was in the specialty community, causing some feeling of displacement by the general practitioners. For example, the general practitioners did not have a separate section that met in the hospital. As a consequence, to have a voice in the hospital staff, they attended surgery or medicine department meetings. That left them feeling out of the mainstream in the medical staff. Thus, with this as a background and the board of the CTMF made up predominantly of doctors in specialty practices, there was some element of natural schism and certainly some potential friction.[66]

There was enough tension in the process of planning and moving toward construction of the building that a number of the family practice doctors considered gathering sufficient numbers/votes at an upcoming general Travis County Medical Society meeting to vote the members of the CTMF board out and to restructure the CTMF board. Sufficient meetings and negotiations were carried out to avoid that disruptive approach and the community returned to working together to complete the building project. I believe Marshal Cothran's diplomatic personality played a major role in that process. The Blackstock clinic was built at 4614 N. I-35 and occupied in 1991. It provided satisfactory working space and location for use over the next ten years. The service remained in that building until a couple of years after Seton assumed the management of Brackenridge in 1995 and the training program in

1998. The Blackstock clinic was moved to the Brackenridge Professional Building immediately next to the hospital. The idea presented by Seton was that this would place the residents close to the hospital and closer to the hospital care in which the residents were engaged. It would consolidate the residency programs in a more central location relative to the other services. There was some discontent about giving up their own building. The building was eventually leased to the City for a clinic and became the David Powell clinic for HIV/AIDs treatment.

Dr. Mathis Blackstock grew up in Austin and completed high school here. He attended the University of Texas, Austin for his undergraduate years and then the University of Texas Medical Branch in Galveston and graduated in 1948. He practiced in Ganado, Texas for four months before starting his internship year and a year of Obstetrics and Gynecology at Hermann Hospital in Houston. He was married after completing his internship year. That was followed by two years of general practice residency in Denver, Colorado, interrupted by two years in the Navy during the Korean War. On completing his residency, he opened a practice in Kerrville, Texas. Although he described it as a wonderful place to practice, as he had Ganado, Texas, he took the opportunity to cover the practice of Dr. Sig Hayes in Austin while Dr. Hayes was serving two years, 1955 and 1956, in the National Guard. Following those two years, Dr. Blackstock joined Dr. Hayes' practice and they remained together until 1974. He did not return to Kerville. In 1974, Dr. Hayes moved to Bertram and Dr. Blackstock started working at the Rosewood Zaragosa Clinic. This was to be followed by his association with the Family Practice residency program until 2012.

Dr. Johnson talked with Dr. Blackstock in 1978, asking him to consider becoming an associate director of the Family Practice program. Dr. Blackstock had been taking interns and residents into his private office for years as preceptors, and had enjoyed the teaching experience. He had also worked in the Rosewood Zaragosa Clinic, after leaving private practice in 1974 when Dr. Hayes left. He chose to take the job, working in both of the Rosewood Zaragosa clinic in east Austin in the mornings with residents and the Family Health Center in the afternoons. Dr. Johnson would go from the Family Health Center in the morning to his private practice office in the afternoons.[61]

In time, Dr. Johnson became involved with managed care programs and left the teaching program to be associated with The Texas Health

Plan. This was a managed health plan with doctors of the Travis County Medical Society as members. This was to be a closed health panel that would compete with managed care plans form the various insurance companies. Following Dr. Johnson's tenure, Dr. David Wright became the medical director of the Family Practice department for five to six years.

David Wright had come to the community as a VISTA volunteer and served in a south Austin clinic where Dr. Blackstock, Dr. Ben White and others served low-income patients. He also met and later married, Sheri, another volunteer working at the clinic. He was encouraged to go to medical school and attended UTMB. He was so impressed by Dr. Blackstock and the medicine in Austin that he spent some of his third year and about seventy percent of his fourth year in Austin, mostly at Brackenridge. He was particularly interested in how physicians could be in touch with their patients and ultimately affect the community in which they practiced. He also observed the level of involvement and dedication between departments in the medical community and felt he might be able to make a contribution to that area of medicine in Austin. On returning to Austin Dr. Wright completed his family practice residency and then joined the faculty. He was completely devoted to Dr. Blackstock and chose to emulate his approach to practice and to be as complete a doctor as possible. He became quite involved with the treatment of AIDS patients in the early 1980s as that disease was new and of great concern as a threat to patients and the medical community. Following his tenure as medical director he has continued in the teaching program remaining true to his goal of being a complete clinical doctor and teacher.[67]

In one of our recent conversations, he noted that he felt as if he was much more on his own in the practice of medicine and teaching. Dr. Blackstock, Dr. Bain, Dr. Ben White and others had passed away. Many others, including me, as a consultant and an instructor for the residents, had retired and were not available for consultations, as we had been for years. This thought mirrored my own thinking some twenty years earlier as my mentors had gradually left the scene and I was left wondering, as in the Pete Seeger song "Where have all the flowers gone," here condensed:

Where have all the flowers (mentors) gone?
Young girls picked them everyone.
Where have all the young girls gone?
Gone to young men every one.
Where have all the young men gone?
Gone for soldiers every one.
Where have all the soldiers gone?
Gone to graveyards every one....

Well, they had all gone to retirement, other fields or to the graveyards under the flowers every one. It is a sobering realization that you may have become a senior mentor and that others are depending on you for information and direction.

Returning to our narrative, following Dr. Wright's leadership, Dr. Walter "Dick" Leverich, a 1986 graduate of the University of Texas at San Antonio became the interim medical director. He had completed his family practice residency in Austin. He spent two years as director and then moved to full time private practice in northwest Austin. His directorship was followed by that of Dr. Jim Knale, Dr. Blackstock as interim director, and then Dr. Cynthia Brinson. Dr. Brinson met her husband in Austin and then went to Texas Tech University Medical School, graduating in 1990. She left her husband working in Austin. She returned to Austin for her family practice residency, joined the faculty in 1994 and became interim director in 1996 and director from 1998-99. I had the pleasure of meeting her in 1991, when she spent her orthopedic rotation as a resident in our office. She enjoyed patient care and teaching but after Seton Hospitals took over the teaching program from CTMF in 1998, they seemed to want an administrative director who would spend much of the day in meetings or with paper work. That was not to her liking so she joined the Red River Family Practice group in 1999, where she has remained. She was hired by Seton in 2012 to work one day a week on curriculum.[68]

It should be noted that in the 1970s there were 8-10 residents rotating through the Family Practice section. At the end of Dr. Brinson's tenure there were 21 residents rotating through Family Practice clinics; orthopedics; intensive care unit; pediatric outpatient clinic; community medicine; urology; ear, nose, and throat; dermatology; renal; cardiology; neurology; rural medicine; obstetrics and gynecology; gastroenterology; and emergency room. All of this involved different rotations for each resident and a different program for first, second and third year residents. It was time consuming to keeping all the services satisfied with the rotations, to have consultants available, and to keep the program accredited. There have been twelve clinical directors of the Family Practice service from 1974 to the present. This appears to reflect a program run by community doctors, many of whom had private practices or other responsibilities in additions to the responsibilities of the service. It is a testament to those individuals who have been willing to sacrifice much time to ensure the encouragement and training of future doctors of the community in family practice.

In the late 1980's and into the 1990's there was a clear evolution of the department relative to community family practice doctors helping with the clinics and providing rotations for residents through their offices. Part of the Medicare payments to hospitals with training programs is payment for patient care. Medicare placed requirements/strings on those payments based on doctor visits to the patients. It was no longer possible for the staff doctor to just initial the resident's notes. The staff doctor had to make a significant entry into the chart to document patient visits and resident teaching. This resulted in a significant increase in the time commitment for seeing patients with the residents. It was noted that, although some doctors had agreed to cover the clinics, their office demands interfered with their actually coming to help the residents. Therefore some of the clinics weren't covered and the residents were seeing patients by themselves. By the early 1990's it became necessary to hire full or part time faculty to cover the clinic responsibilities. The era of community doctors providing the bulk of the teaching had come to an end and CTMF began a new era in the teaching program, namely paid faculty to cover the teaching.

Still, as part of the training, many private doctors agreed to take the residents into their offices for an experience with private practice settings. Neurologists, dermatologists, pediatricians, urologists, various internal medicine subspecialties, ophthalmologists, ear, nose and throat specialists and orthopedists, among others, were willing to take residents into their offices for a month at a time. As an example, our office, The Austin Bone and Joint Clinic, had about seventy-five residents rotate through our office from 1989 through 2006, when I retired. These included both family practice and internal medicine residents. We also had several interns who spent a month at a time back in the early 1970 before and just after CTMF started. (A complete list of those residents is in the Appendix).

When the residents were rotating though the various private offices they did not have hospital responsibilities. They would come daily to the private practices and observe the patients and the office procedures that were involved. In our office, we would have them see new patients first, take a history, do an examination and present their findings to us. Meanwhile, we might have time to see other patients. After the presentation, we would review the history with the patient and check the exam. We would read x-rays together, when available, and then formulate a treatment plan. It was important to us that the resident come up with their own plan and go through the thought process of what to do with or for the patient. Hopefully, in our office, we would have a splint or cast to change or a new one to apply. This technique would be valuable to them in their future practice. We would get the resident to do as much of that procedure as was practical. I suspect that the same approach was available in the other specialty offices.

Of course, the surgery, obstetrics, pediatric and internal medicine services had a great deal of contact with residents in the hospital. The specialty doctors had much less contact, since their hospital patients were not assigned to the resident staff. As general surgeons and orthopedic surgeons we spent our lives in the emergency room. On average the general surgeons would be called to the ER about 110-115 times each month and the orthopedists on call would be called roughly 100-105 times. In the ER we would come in contact with the residents. If there was a resident also in the ER and they were not terribly busy, they might be enticed into looking at our patients as well. The two most frequent patients seen by the orthopedists were automobile accident victims and children with fractures. The automobile accident patients were most often complicated cases with long bone fractures or multiple injuries. Those were not the type of patients the family practice doctors were going to see in their future. Children, with simple fractures, would definitely be something they would see in their future practices and for which they needed experience.

In managing these patients we would get our uncomplicated patients out of the noisy ER and moved to the cast room, near the operating room suite. There we could have our own quiet area to work and also have help from the nursing staff from the OR. The parents could come along to provide reassurance and aid the child's comfort. The residents could come with us, observe the routine of making the child and parents comfortable, obtaining help from the hospital staff, be involved with the communication process, and finally see the technical process of setting a fracture. Once we were in the quiet of the cast room, the child was much more comfortable and generally not so frightened. The fracture pain would have settled. After explaining the procedure to the child, a local injection of novocaine/lidocaine would be administered into the local blood around the fracture, pain would completely resolve, the reduction would be done and the splint applied. This procedure was extremely common and the procedure of setting the bone quite routine. It was hoped that the family would be comfortable, but also the resident could see that it could be a calm procedure with which they could deal in the future. They would certainly have similar patients in their offices, especially in more rural settings. Most of the fractures with which they would be involved would be non-displaced, or not out of alignment, and would only require a splint, with which they would be completely comfortable.

One of the residents who rotated through our office was Dr. Tom Zavaleta. He attended the University of Texas Medical School in San Antonio, having graduated in 1974. He did his first year of pediatric residency in San Antonio and then transferred to Austin, ultimately completing his chief residency year in 1978. At that time the nursery was in the old red brick building facing IH-35. Karen Teel was the director and he remembered her as a wonderful teacher. Many of the community pediatricians were the attending at the time. He joined the private practice of the Austin Children's Clinic for his first years in practice and then moved to Austin Regional Clinic where he practiced for a number of years. In his pediatric practice, a number of his patient's parents asked if he would be their primary doctor, although that was not practical. In 1998 he decided to return to the training program, this time to family practice. With his twenty years of pediatric practice he did not have to repeat any pediatric rotation. As with many residents he spent a month in our office, learning orthopedics, which would be helpful on returning to a general practice setting. He told me at the time that he thought he might semi-retire in a few years, move to Ruidoso, New Mexico, and open a small practice. That part of his plan never materialized. During his rotation with us he learned a bit more anatomy, how to care for back pain, shoulder and knee problems, and the art of injecting larger joints, using techniques to minimize pain. Back pain and joint aches are surprisingly common complaints in general practice patients and he later stated he used that information regularly. After completing that training he returned to Austin Regional Clinic office until 2010, when he switched to the Wellmed geriatric office. The flexibility of the smaller community based Brackenridge training program seemed to have fit his circumstances much better than a large academic program.[56]

Following Dr. Brinson's tenure in 1999, Dr. Kavle became the director for a year. He left to pursue other interests, one of which was to be come involved with Hospice Austin. Dr. Dana Sprute, a graduate of the Brackenridge family practice program, who had been working with Dr. Brinson, took over as interim director. Dr. Russell Thomas was then hired as permanent director of the department. He was originally from Eagle Lake, Texas where his father was a doctor. During his time as director, his father passed away. Dr. Thomas felt the draw of his small hometown community and, as his father was the only doctor in town, he was pulled back home to take over the practice there. Dr. Sprute again became interim director.

Dr. Sam Adkins was next in line and headed the department for 6 years, from 2003 to 2009. He was originally from North Carolina; he left in 2009 to return to North Carolina to work for the North Carolina Health Systems in the area of health information. It was during his administration that the decision was made to move the Family Medicine residents that had been rotating at St. David's back to Brackenridge. In the past there had been some difficulty dividing the patients between Internal Medicine and Family Medicine. Dr. Adkins felt that problem could be overcome and he wanted much more presence of the Family Medicine department at Brackenridge.

When Dr. Adkins left for North Carolina, Dr. Dana Sprute was named the program director, this time as full time director. She had attended the University of Texas Medical School at San Antonio and graduated in 1993. She then started her family medicine residency at Brackenridge and completed it in 1996. Her first job was to work for the Austin Diagnostic Clinic at a South Austin clinic with Dr. David Carter and Dr. David Joseph. She had worked there for two years when a faculty position and funding became available at Brackenridge in

1998. Dr. Brinson asked her to join the faculty when her contract was completed with ADC. She was interim medical director twice before being asked to become the full time director in 2009. Dr. Carter and Dr. Joseph have remained colleagues as they work part-time as clinical faculty.[69]

In the mid 1990's there were approximately twenty-one residents and that number has remained rather stable to the present. I note that there are twenty-one residents in the program for the 2015-16 year; seven are male and fourteen are female. Medical students from UTMB take much of their core third-year curriculum in Austin, adding to the teaching load. As of 2015 there were eight faculty working in the program with four full-time members. Dr. Kelly Alberda and Dr. Lisa Clemons are in charge of the family medicine obstetrics section, Dr. Swati Avashia the pediatric section, Dr. Terrell Benold office surgery, and Dr. David Wright clinical teaching and faculty development. In addition, there are faculty positions in psychology, pharmacy and social work.

Funding for the program comes through Seton, the Texas Higher Education Coordinating Board, Medicare and Medicaid payments and some insurance plans.

As of January, 2015, the program is included in the department of Population Health at the University of Texas at Austin Dell Medical School. That department is charged with improving the overall health of the people of Travis County, a huge undertaking. Dr. William Tierney is the chairman of that department with the rather high calling of disseminating new models of care to improve outcomes, improve health information (medical records) tools, improve occupational health, and some possible outreach to international programs.[70]

The outpatient clinic service for family medicine remains in the Brackenridge Professional Office building where it has functioned since leaving the Blackstock Clinic. The family practice clinic, still called the Blackstock Clinic, has now achieved the status of a Federally Qualified Health Clinic (FQHC). With that status there is another source of revenue and the payments from Medicare are definitely improved. With that status also comes a long string of requirements, red tape and interruptions that are necessary to maintain their standing for federal support. There are strict reporting requirements regarding follow up of chronic illness so that the central authorities can collect statistics and maintain controls in health care. There are also some peculiar rules regarding what can be done in the clinic. An administrative individual entered the clinic one day and removed the cast cart, with all the splinting material and the cast saw. When asked why that was done, even thought it was used regularly in patient care, the response was that all similar clinics do not have doctors that are trained in casting, so none of the clinics can use that equipment. For a similar reason, all of the off-the-shelf wrist splints were removed, again because all members might not be trained in their use. The microscopes were removed one day as they might be construed as instruments of a laboratory service for which a financial charge could be made. They were actually used for training when the residents might look at urine or vaginal samples. Finally they removed all the drug samples as inappropriate for use in the clinic as they had not been placed in the inventory by the pharmacy.

Medical records remain an issue in this department. The check box system of collecting medical information for electronic medical records has significant deficiencies in the nuances of medical histories. Dr. Wright has a lot of concern about the use of those tools for training medical students who will be rotating through the service. Collecting medically relevant information by utilizing a "check the box" system is a vastly different process, as compared to bringing that list up in your own mind, collecting the data, establishing priorities, and then using that information in a differential diagnosis and treatment plan.[67,69]

The Family Medicine section has weathered several storms over the years with thirteen different program directors, challenges with accreditation early on, moving from one clinic to another, and maintaining working relationships with a large number of private practitioners; however it has continued to attract quality residents, many of whom have stayed in Austin for their private practices and added value to the medical community.

Psychiatry Department

Psychiatry and psychiatric treatment, especially in the public domain, seems to get the short end of the straw when it comes to money and recognition. I assume that is because everyone thinks they may get appendicitis, break an arm, or get pregnant and need hospitalization. They certainly don't think they are going to be mentally ill, so they are less willing to support mental treatment institutions. Mental illness has a fear factor that definitely puts people off when discussing health care. On the other hand, the first hospital in America was in Williamsburg, Virginia and was a mental hospital.

Placing the discussion of the psychiatric department toward the end of our writing has little to do with basic importance; that has more to do with how quiet that program seemed to the general medical community. It was not primarily centered at Brackenridge or other acute care hospitals and was not included in the CTMF or AMEP oversight until recently.

In our history in Austin, the first truly organized independent residency program in the City was started at the Austin State Hospital on Guadalupe Street, (formerly Asylum Road), the mental facility, in about 1955. The residency was supported by the State through the hospital and with money from the legislature under the State Department of Mental Health and Mental Retardation (MHMR). The program was directed by Dr. Hoerster who was also the superintendent of the State Hospital. The primary inpatient treatment area was established at the Austin State Hospital, one of several State mental facilities. There was no direct arrangement for consultations to be provided at Brackenridge or the other acute care hospitals. Psychiatric patients were transferred from acute care facilities all over the state and evaluated by the residents and staff to see if the admission was appropriate.

In 1962, Dr. Beverly Sutton came to Austin because her husband was appointed to the faculty of the University of Texas with his PhD in Genetics. She had obtained her medical degree from the University of Michigan and then had completed a one-year internship, two years of pediatric residency and two years of child psychiatry, also at Michigan. It was quite unusual for a resident to complete child psychiatry before doing adult psychiatric training but she was interested in child psychiatry all along. She did the pediatric medical residency so that she would be prepared if a presumed psychiatric illness was really an illness of retardation or some other medical condition.

She was interviewed by Dr. Hoester for the residency in adult psychiatry. He asked her what she could do for the program here. She said she would do an "honest days work" and with her training in child psychiatry would want to work with that program as well. After completing her two years of adult psychiatry residency, she joined the staff and began to develop a child psychiatry department. She found that the children were all mixed in with the adult patients on the resident floors. The children would take advantage of the adults and ask for treats and would even have the adults offer them cigarettes. The adults were very generous with the children, but it was, of course, a dangerous situation. She reviewed 155 children and found a large number with mental retardation rather than a psychiatric diagnosis. There were some thirty different developmental conditions the children had that needed to be separated from the mental illness categories. These children were discharged back home with the cooperation of the judge from the county from which they had been admitted. The mentally ill boys were then separated from the men's unit. It required a certain amount of disciplining of the staff to keep the children off the adult unit where they had been spoiled by adult patients in the past. The girls remained on the women's unit for the time being. The residents were involved with this change and gained important experience, as they would eventually run into these problems wherever they ultimately practiced.

In 1971, with the help of Hill Burton federal funds, a children's building was constructed north of 45th Street, next to the Child Guidance center. There had been no schooling provided for the children, so Dr.

Sutton got the Austin Independent School District involved. They provided new teachers who were added to other volunteer staff of social workers, psychologists, and an analyst. The analyst, Joe Wakefield, volunteered to lecture for years and coordinated his transference and defense topics with Dr. Sutton's child development lectures. Under State law, the volunteers were protected from law suits that might arise from anything that happened during their association with the mental patients.

Dr. Sutton, meanwhile, continued her research into the biochemical and genetic implications of mental illness and child development. Her husband proved to be a rich source of information regarding some of the genetic disorders that would present themselves in the symptoms of her patients. It was said that during her tenure, she had obtained about $4.2 million from federal grants for her research with the addition of funds from the Hard Foundation.

As Dr. Sutton was the director of the child psychiatry division for many years, the adult section was led in turn by Dr. Hoerster, Dr. Anthony Rousos, Dr. Joe Zachariah, Dr. Ed Penny, and Dr. Larry Hauser (acting director). Dr. Hauser was instrumental in starting a program, in 1985, in which the residents would provide consultative services to Brackenridge and other hospitals in the community. This filled a real need in the acute care facilities where, particularly, the internal medicine doctors felt they needed help for patients with psychiatric illnesses. In addition to the consult service, Dr. Hauser provided psychosomatic services and instruction to the residents.

The residency program continued to be supported through MHMR until 2003 when the State of Texas cut the funding for training, leaving the program without resources. The legislature decided that they would provide money for mental health services but not for training. This meant that the residency program would need to find funding or positions for the residents. After almost 50 years of stable support, the legislature removed that stability. Dr. Sutton, who was at that time managing both the adult and children's services, had to scramble; she contacted programs all over the state to secure new positions for all of the residents. At about that time, Dr. Sutton talked to Dr. Jim Lindsey about the possibility that Seton and the Austin Medical Education Program (AMEP) might take the residency under its wing with the other residency services. As a result of those discussions, the General

Psychiatry and the Child and Adolescent Psychiatry Residency program joined the Austin Medical education program (AMEP), gained funding through that support system, and was able to keep all their resident positions. With the State no longer supporting the residency, the program moved to Shoal Creek Hospital, the private mental health facility located on Shoal Creek between 34th and 38th streets. The children's program remained at the building on 45th Street. The Austin State hospital hired additional doctors to cover the patient care that had been provided by the residents. In 2004, with the move to Shoal Creek, the adult program came under the directorship of Dr. Kari Wolf who was also the director of the Seton Mind Institute. Under AMEP, the program was able to add new faculty, increase the number of residents from 16 to 24, and work collaboratively with public mental health systems, the UT college of Education, and many private physicians in the community. Dr. Sutton retired in 2010 and the directorship was then taken on by Dr. Jane Rippinger-Sueler. During the years of independent training there were several associate/assistant directors including Dr. Marjorie Lawlis, Dr. Kira Carey, Dr. Katherine Miller and Dr. Jay Allen Davis.[71]

As of 2015 the program was being absorbed into the department of the Dell Medical School and a full time director had not been selected.

Pathology

In the earlier part of this book, we noted that Dr. Dan Queen was the head of the pathology department. He had started having weekly pathology conferences for the interns in the late 1950s. Dr. Jimmy Harrod was giving gynecological pathology conferences. In the early 1960s Dr. Queen also took on the role of part time director of the internship training program. Dr. Queen accepted an offer to become the head of pathology at the new Methodist hospital in San Antonio. Dr. Atys Da Silva, an associate, then became the head of pathology at Brackenridge and the acting director of the training program. He remained in that position until Dr. Pape became acting director of the training program in 1963. The pathology department had started taking on trainees as residents and had become accredited by the American Medical Association in those years under the supervision of Dr. Da Silva. He was a remarkable individual who guided and molded the pathology section and encouraged the development of the pathology residency. He had done his medical school training in his home country of Brazil and then his pathology in Indiana. Interestingly, he maintained a significant relationship with doctors in Brazil and was regularly sent pathological specimens for consultation from several different cities in Brazil. He was very interested in personal service as a consultant and encouraged that in his colleagues. 1964, Dr. James Spidle became the first pathology resident. He completed his residency in 1968 and stayed on at Brackenridge in the department for many years. Dr. Charles D. Bell took one year in 1973-74. He returned to family practice in south Texas.

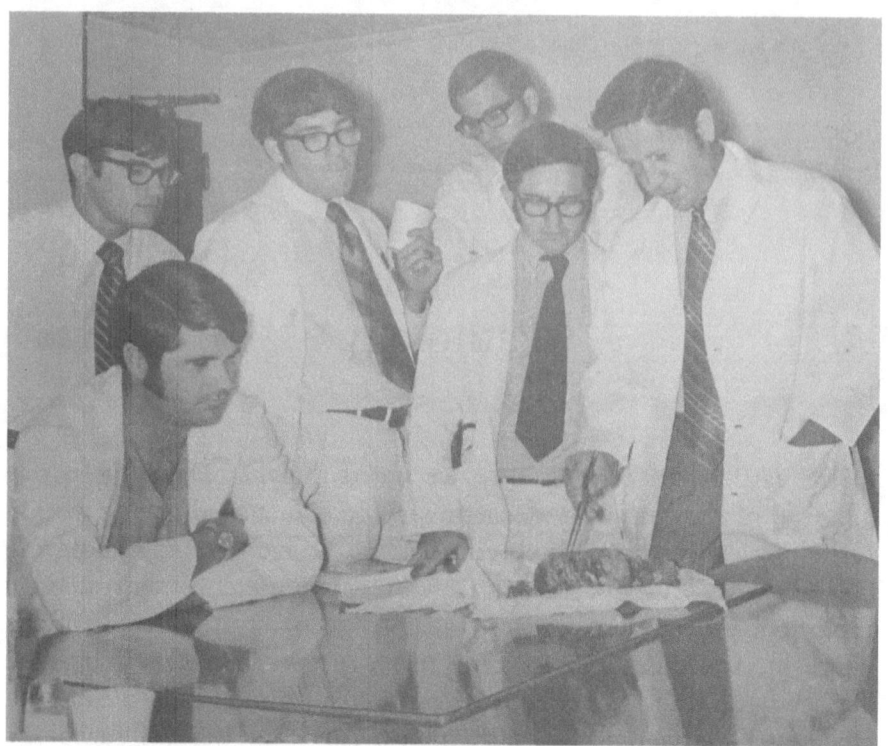

Pathology teaching session. Dr. Spidle on the right. Dr. John Boyd, left, Dr. Bobby Maddor, behind, Dr. Dan Cravey, tallest behind.

Dr. Donald Parsons joined the department as a staff pathologist in 1974, having completed his residency at Fitzsimons Army Hospital in Denver.[72] Dr. William Reitmeyer and Dr. Paul LeBourgouis completed their four-year programs in 1979 under Drs. Da Silva, Spidle, Parsons and McClurg. Dr. McClurg joined the department after completing her pathology residency in Dallas. The residents spent most of their time looking at pathological specimens in the lab, consulting with physicians on the floors, supervising the laboratory for blood testing, and doing a number of autopsies. Dr. Reitmeyer does remember that some of the deceased were from drowning in Lake Austin. An autopsy has been required in the State of Texas when ordered by the justice of the peace as part of the investigation of a death. Initially there was no medical examiner in Austin but, during the period of Dr. Reitmeyer's residency, Dr. Robert Buckland was hired as medical examiner. The medical examiner would then complete the autopsies formerly done by the pathology department. Dr. Reitmeyer joined the department following his residency and remained in that position until 1989. The Children's Hospital was being built at that time and he chose to take an additional year of fellowship in children's pathology with Dr. Bruce Beckwist. He returned to Brackenridge and covered the increasing demand for pathology at Children's. In 2003 he started consulting at the Austin Diagnostic Clinic and then, in 2007, joined a new group that provided consultation at Seton, Seton Cedar Park and Harker Heights.[73]

Dr. Parsons remained with the department until 1990 when he joined the pathology department at the Central Texas Medical Center in San Marcos.[72] Dr. Randy Ralph did a three-years residency from 1979 through 1982.

Dr. Suzanna Dana started her residency in 1979 at Baylor Hospital in Dallas after finishing medical school. After one year she married a man whose business was in Austin and she transferred to Brackenridge. She thought leaving Dallas might be a significant compromise but found the program in Austin very enjoyable, almost like being part of the staff. She found Drs. Da Silva, Parsons, Reitmeyer, and Phil Collins most helpful. She was interested in forensic pathology so she was more interested in doing autopsies than the rest of the staff. On completing three years in Austin in 1983, plus the one in Dallas, she was contacted by Dr. Vincent Dimaio in San Antonio who was looking for a resident to do a year in forensic pathology. This was right down her alley and she took that opportunity. After her time with Dr. Dimaio, she became a medical examiner in San Antonio, Bexar County. She later worked in Travis County, until 2006, and then formed her own private practice to perform forensic pathology. She and Dr. Randy Ralph were the last residents to complete full residencies at Brackenridge.[74]

In 1982-83 Dr. Robert S. Zirl and Dr. Robert S. Hanes started their first year as residents. Following them was Dr. Cory Jammal as first-year in 1983-84. Dr. Edward Randy Eckert was a first-year in 1984 and was listed as a third year, completing December 31st, 1986.

The program had been run and supported by the group of pathologists in the department, the Austin Pathology Associates. Amazingly they had paid the salaries of the residents for many years. This is the only program of which I am aware that was supported financially by the doctors who managed the program. Dr. Phillip Collins became the director of pathology training when he joined the practice after completing his residency at UT Southwestern in Dallas in 1981. The program eventually joined with the CTMF organization. CTMF provided administrative functions and contributed about fifty percent of the funding of the resident salaries. The pathologists provided all of the teaching, including direct supervision and multiple pathology conferences for the pathology residents as well as conferences for the other services such as surgery, medicine, pediatrics, obstetrics, and others. In contrast to other departments, all of the actions of the pathology residents were required to be one hundred percent supervised. That meant that no pathology report was sent out without review by the staff and therefore there was no work reduction by the assistance of the residents efforts. As insurance reimbursement changed and tightened, it was difficult to maintain the time spent with residents and the workload. The program therefore approached CTMF to ask for funds to pay all of the residents stipends and not just part. As CTMF may not have understood the one hundred percent supervision required of the residents, they declined to cover all of those costs. As a consequence, the pathologists decided to close the residency program as too costly. Many smaller programs across the country were also closing as they had difficulty competing with university programs in recruiting residents. Thus, with the conclusion of the program, Dr. Zirl found a position in Houston and Dr. Randy Eckert left in December of 1986 to complete his final two years at Tulane in New Orleans. Dr. Eckert eventually returned to Austin to join the Austin Pathological Associates group.[75]

The pathology department, therefore, although the second accredited program available in Austin, is the only one to be abandoned as not practical to continue. It is a testament to Dr. Da Silva, and later his partners, that it was looked upon so favorably and lasted twenty-five years.

Transitional years of the early 21st Century

A number of forces over the years have contributed to changes in the training program and to Brackenridge Hospital. The number of community doctors who have been committed to serving Brackenridge and its mission has varied from time to time but generally has been surprisingly strong. The complexities introduced by payers for medical services has become much more intense and that has demanded additional physician time for managing their practices, thus limiting discretionary time. The discounting of fees by the payers has caused doctors to say they "gave at the office" and they are therefore less likely to give also at the hospitals. As the other community hospitals got bigger and provided more services, loyalties to those institutions shifted. As an example, Brackenridge was the place where most orthopedic surgery was performed and where cardiovascular surgery started in Austin. With time, those services expanded to other hospitals and, thus, shifted talent away from Brackenridge. With larger institutions and more street traffic, there was less need or desire to "cover multiple hospitals," so many doctors chose to provide their time at one place. When doctors began to be paid for covering emergency rooms, and that spread to other hospitals, there was, clearly, a different approach to call assignments. And as more and more paid faculty were hired for the teaching staff, more community doctors shifted away from covering Brackenridge. The program needed more assurance of coverage for clinics and inpatients than the community doctors could or would provide on a regular basis. Medicare and other payers demanded that staff doctors spend more time, making it harder for volunteer staff to teach and maintain a private practice. The creation of CTMF changed the formula a great deal and started it on its way toward a larger organization. Psychologically, it made the training programs feel more like an "institutional" entity and less a community cooperative responsibility.

It is hard to emphasize enough how important to the process the changes in payments for medical care by insurer were. The largest single payer, Medicare, became the uncertain force with which to be reckoned. Medicare basically paid fee for service for the first fifteen to twenty years (after 1968) and then changed their method to a managed care model. They also used a formula of Diagnosis Related Groups, (DRGs) to bundle payments. This, in effect, lowered fees significantly from traditional relative values scales. The private insurance companies developed Health Maintenance Organizations, formed partnerships or just merged and offered negotiated fees. Fees for Medicare and from private insurers were actually not negotiated but were offered as "take it or leave it" reduced payments. Medicare arbitrarily reduced their fees and the private insurance companies followed suit, chasing the lowest fees that would not alienate doctors. This created great uncertainty in both private offices and hospitals, at least enough to cause some to stop participating in charitable work altogether. Hospitals needed to make sure they would be able to meet their expenses. As many were non-profit organizations, they did not have enormous reserves to cover shortfalls. As a result, there was a bit of a scramble to join with other organizations to improve their market share, diversify and enlarge their geographic draw of patients, improve their negotiating position with insurance companies by covering these larger geographic areas, and, bottom line, improve their cash positions.

St. David's hospital had a long history of association with Brackenridge. They were involved with the program for family practice residents, providing hospital rotations in which residents would see patients and gain additional experience. They had a similar mission to serve the needy and had an established program to provide obstetrics services to expectant mothers on Medicaid and to take care of the higher number of premature infants in that group of patients. And the neonatologists worked both at Brackenridge and St. David's caring for these at risk newborns. As a consequence, St. David's first choice for an association with another hospital was to approach Brackenridge in the early 1990's to explore the possibility of working more closely together.

There were several meetings that also included public input to explore these ideas. There were quite a few unknowns and it is possible that support by the pediatricians to maintain a centralized pediatric hospital at Brackenridge became a factor, leading to a loss of momentum for that partnership. St. David's even approached Seton Hospital, but because the two hospitals covered such a large proportion of patients in the city, it was likely that the Justice Department would not look at the possibility of loss of competitiveness favorably. St. David's ultimately entered into an agreement with the Hospital Corporation of America (HCA) in 1996 to manage their ever-enlarging hospital system.[76]

The next large-scale change occurred when Seton elected to take over management of Brackenridge from the City in 1995 and then incorporate the training program under that umbrella on March 31, 1998. This part of the story goes back a few years to pick up the main characters. Dr. James O. Lindsey went to Harvard undergraduate where one of his classmates was Bruce Malone, later an orthopedic surgeon in our practice in Austin. Dr. Lindsey then attended medical school at Washington University in St. Louis, completing his studies in 1969. That was followed by an internal medicine and pulmonary residency before he came to Austin in 1976. He joined the practice of the Capital Medical Clinic that had its offices in Medical Park Towers, next to the Seton main hospital. During that period, he was appointed to be a member of the board of the Central Texas Medical Foundation and was its president for two of those years. After twelve years in private practice he found that he enjoyed the administrative side of medicine and joined the staff at Seton Hospital as the Medical Director in 1989. It was in that general period of time that several of the hospitals hired doctors to become medical directors to oversee credentialing, quality care, infectious disease, and the various department committees. This put a medical face on the complex business of running a large hospital. Later in time, Dr. Lindley would manage the administrative functions for the training program when Seton took over that area. It was not long after that that the Chief Executive Officer (CEO) of Seton hospital, Judy Smith, took a job opportunity in Michigan and left Seton. It was also at that time that Seton North West hospital opened, increasing management complexities. With the departure of Judy Smith, a search firm was hired to look for a new CEO. A former Chief Operating Officer, Mr. Charles J. Barnett, from Virginia, was hired and arrived in

1993. Mr. Barnet felt that to be a successful medical facility they need to form a network of several hospitals. This was to follow a national trend in hospital consolidations and acquisitions, including St. David's, as noted above.

Within the first couple of years of Mr. Barnett's tenure, discussions were held with the Austin Diagnostic Clinic, a large multispecialty clinic, to build a joint hospital in north Austin. Ultimately, that partnership did not come to fruition and Austin Diagnostic Clinic built the hospital in partnership with the Hospital Corporation of America (HCA) in 1995. That hospital joined the St. David's system in 2000.

With the long history of charitable care under the Sisters of Charity, Mr. Barnett looked at enlarging the Seton network of hospitals by offering to manage Brackenridge for the City of Austin.

As the City was ambivalent about continuing the management of Brackenridge they had explored multiple alternatives over the past several years. A significant incentive for Seton to consider this partnership included the reality of having the Children's Hospital as part of that package. Insurance companies look at hospitals as service units with which they may have to negotiate; having a large pediatric service would provide a significant competitive edge to Seton's service line. There were some who said that Seton would take over the management of Brackenridge and would add Children's hospital for an extra dollar. What a deal! And everyone knew that Brackenridge would most likely lose money but the Children's Hospital would make money. Children's health care is, by and large, reasonably well funded with private insurance, Medicaid, Aid to Families with Dependent Children (AFDC), and the Children's Health Insurance Program (CHIP). In addition, children's charities tend to garner much larger contributions from the public.

In 1995, Seton negotiated a contract with the City to take over management of Brackenridge Hospital. That would entail multiple complexities: of money exchange; staffing; and, one of the more complex situations, that of having a Catholic organization manage women's health care involving abortions, contraceptive care and tubal ligations. Much of that has been discussed under the Obstetrics and Gynecological service of the teaching program. I was on the Brackenridge Board, as past president of the medical staff, in 1995 when the last meeting of the board was held and the meeting adjourned. It was an interesting little moment in a long history.

Seton then negotiated with the Travis County Medical Society to take over management of the training program in 1998. The Medical Society had become increasingly nervous about their financial arrangement with the City to support the training program. As a non-profit organization, they did not have the financial reserves to deal with the inconsistencies or shortfalls in the budget if the City funding was not promptly paid. Thus, this created the impetus to make arrangements with Seton.

With the acquisition of Brackenridge, the Children's Hospital, and the training program, Seton has changed the landscape of medicine in Austin more that any other single action in its history, except for, perhaps, the original opening of Brackenridge.

As part of the mandated function of managing Brackenridge Hospital, Seton took on the responsibility of providing charity care to patients in the city and ultimately to surrounding counties because of the very active emergency room. With time, it was felt that the teaching program would provide care for indigent patients with less cost than other alternatives. Soon after Seton taking over the training program it became starkly apparent that running a complex training program with a growing teaching faculty, residency house staff, office support staff for the faculty, accreditation requirements, and many details, was well beyond the experience of the Seton staff. Dr. Jim Lindsey became the DIO, (designated institutional officer) who would be responsible, with the department heads, for maintaining the many requirements to make sure that the programs remained accredited. But more experienced help was going to be required to make sure that things would run smoothly.

It was around 2002 that Seton began looking for assistance in managing the training program. It was also about this time that our old partner in training, UTMB, was working through the possibilities of creating a satellite campus in Austin for the medical school. They had sent students to Austin since the 1970's and were interested in sending more students, as well as surgery and obstetrics residents. Austin needed their experience in running a program and a DIO to assist in the implementation of programs to maintain accreditation and improved curriculum. Included in those negotiations was the subject of creating a regional medical center more closely associated with Galveston. As this arrangement matured, there would be provision for more third year medical school students and ultimately fourth year students to rotate to Austin. Thus, in 2005, an arrangement was agreed upon where by UTMB would become the managing partner and sponsor of the Graduate Medical Education program at what was now the University Medical Center at Brackenridge. It was under this sponsorship that UTMB was to develop the Obstetrics and Gynecologic department as a separate entity from the program in Galveston. They started by entering into the first year matching program for ob./gyn. for 2005. They were also instrumental in developing the neurology section in 2006 and dermatology in 2008. The general surgery department had navigated a number of changes over the years with St. Joseph, Galveston, and the University of Texas at Houston. With the guidance of UTMB, an independent surgery department was initiated with the National Matching Program starting in 2008.[77]

Other factors, outside of Austin, continued to increase complexity and would ultimately have an effect on the various Austin residency services. In 1998 and 1999, the Residency Review Committee of the Accreditation Council for Graduate Medical Education (ACGME) set new requirements for medical students in Internal Medicine. This required a core clerkship. The development for these programs and clearing the hurdles required to keep them accredited increased the need for association with UTMB. The need to meet the changes in curriculum have molded the thinking both at UTMB and Austin.

In the collaborative arrangement there was certainly room for reciprocity with Austin, as UTMB needed patients in obstetrics and gynecology and more patients for student instruction. As Galveston had a limited patient volume, there was a long tradition of UTMB students going elsewhere for clinical patient care experience. When I was in medical school in the early 1960s, we had medical students from Galveston on obstetrics rotation to Houston to gain experience in delivering babies. So, for multiple reasons, both in Galveston and Austin, this new and evolving arrangement would put UTMB in a better position to send students to Austin for clinical experience. Some students were to spend their entire third year in Austin. Ultimately, arrangements were made for fourth-year students as well. The students have continued to come to Austin as recently as 2015. For multiple reasons the arrangements for a regional medical center for UTMB never came to fruition.

As we look at local and outside influences that affected what happened in Austin, the evolution of the Seton Family of Hospitals is important. The sponsoring organization of Seton was the Daughters of Charity of St. Vincent de Paul. In 2010, the several regional organizations, (eastern United States, north and south, with the exception the western region of the United States), came together as Ascension Health, a ministry of the Catholic Church transcending individual sponsoring organizations. It is assumed that this provided a very solid financial organization with the stated objective to "assure the Ascension as a ministry (that) will be sustained and strengthened over time, both with religious and lay persons serving as members."[78] This would be expected to provide a firm financial base for Seton's involvement with a new medical school. It is assumed that this consolidation was consistent with the many consolidations in the health care community in general, driven by financial projections and uncertainties.

As I noted earlier, when discussing of several departments, 2008 was a pivotal year for the University of Texas Medical Branch. Because of multiple factors including finances, Hurricane Ike, and the insular Galveston medical faculty, they withdrew their management and financial support arrangement with Austin. They had been our partner and advisor since the early 1950's and it was difficult to lose that relationship. The Vice Chancellor for Health Affairs of the University of Texas apparently became involved in this decision and facilitated an arrangement with the University of Texas Southwestern Medical School in Dallas to assume the sponsorship relationship with the Austin program. A contract was negotiated and went into effect December 1, 2009.

As part of this arrangement, Dr. Sue Cox in Dallas was approached to become the UT Southwestern Regional Dean of the Austin programs. She was at the time the Associate Dean of Medical Education and the ACGME Designated Institutional Officer at Southwestern. She had oversight over the 94 residency and fellowship programs in Dallas. For two years she commuted weekly to Austin and maintained her responsibilities in Dallas. In 2011 she was offered the position of Regional Dean for the Austin Medical Education Program at the University of Texas at Austin Dell Medical School. She resigned from her position in Dallas and moved to Austin. Subsequently she became the Executive Vice Dean for Academics and Chair of the Medical Education Program. During the time that UT Southwestern helped manage the Austin program, the departments of dermatology, family medicine, general surgery, internal medicine, neurology, obstetrics/gynecology, pediatrics, psychiatry, child and adolescent psychiatry, and the transitional year program have come under that sponsorship. Subsequently, partially in support of the Trauma Center, the Level I Emergency Room, and also in anticipation of the future medical school, additional departments were developed. These services include psychosomatic medicine (2011); emergency medicine; and physical medicine and rehabilitation (2012); pediatric emergency medicine; child neurology; and craniofacial surgery (2013). In 2002 there were approximately 85 residents in the various programs. That increased to 243 by 2015 and it is anticipated that with full capacity of the current accredited programs in 2016, there will be 266 residents in the Austin programs.[79]

It remains to be seen what factors will most profoundly effect medical education and medical practice in the future. In Austin, the impact of a potentially grand medical school nurtured by the University of Texas, Austin, and its large research interest will be profound. The involvement of a creative entrepreneurial surrounding community and the potential collaboration with the University of Texas could be rather impressive. The creation of a new medical campus, which will soon be outgrown physically, will be interesting to watch. We will undoubtedly move Red River Street a couple more times.

Something that could be more of an influence in the future will be the way medicine deals with two significant factors. One is the ever-increasing number of physicians who are on salary. That has been a concern over the past thirty years in Austin. The mobility and productivity of doctors working for minor emergency rooms is one example. It was the observation of some in the process that keeping those doctors motivated and productive could be a problem from time to time. There was a lot of shifting from one job to another, resulting in great difficulty getting those doctors credentialed on insurance panels in a timely fashion and, therefore, getting them paid for their work at the clinics. That has also been a problem at some large multispecialty clinics. I have personally seen differences in productivity between one department and another that created friction in the overall organization in a different city. Whether that will affect a large University Medical campus seems more remote but still a possibility.

The other factor, that could be earth shattering, is the problem with electronic medical records. In its current format it is cumbersome, technically demanding, intrusive in the doctor patient encounter, very time consuming, and is a long way from being portable or communicative with other computer systems, as envisioned by the creators and developers. It seems to be a very large impediment to training, patient care time, portability, flexibility, and doctor satisfaction. Perhaps its most profound weakness is it inability to relate the nuances and emotional input on the part of the doctor in the patient encounter. This type of information is critical to the actual formation of the thought processes that lead to evaluation of priorities, degrees of illness, and perhaps even motivation to chase after the small details that lead to one diagnosis or the other. Our communication through language is the primary essential in patient care. The basic reason for medical records is to communicate our thoughts to others regarding how we came to the conclusions that we did. Language is the tool by which we think. Actually there is some question whether humans think in any real way other than through their language. If that language is broken up into small sound bites "the pain is sharp, dull, achy, intermittent, located low back" it may result in a very different product/idea than the smooth flowing process of normal speech. It remains to be seen how communication, using an electronic medical record, generally collected by a check-lists and "sound bites" can replace the smooth thinking of every-day language.

As noted by Dr. Wright, teaching medical students and residents requires a specific set of tools. The process of collecting patient information in a coherent history and then formulating a list for differential diagnosis is the essence of the diagnostic process. One must create a list of reasonable diagnostic possibilities in ones mind to work with in the process. Actually, it is not a long list in many cases and it has been observed in some studies that many astute diagnosticians go fairly directly to a limited list of possibilities as they formulate their diagnosis. If one has a list of possibilities on a computer, how do you teach medical students and residents to come up with their own list of priorities? It remains to be seen how these issues will be rectified in the teaching process.

The discussion of the several elements in a transition implies that there is an endpoint in that process, or at least some short-term goal to be achieved. In this case, although the "goal" was an unknown in the past, the creation of a medical school has now become that endpoint. With the exception of San Jose, California Austin is one of the largest cities in the United States without a medical school. There have been discussions of creating a medical school here since, at least, the early 1960s. There was some discussion at that time of moving the medical school from Galveston to Austin. That would have been an economic disaster for Galveston. The population of Galveston peaked in 1960 at around 70,000 and has continued to decline since. The plan never progressed very far. For reasons only the politicians know, Austin was not included when several medical schools were created in Texas in the 1960-70's, including the University of Texas at Houston and San Antonio, Texas Tech University and Texas A & M University Medical School.

Creating a Medical School

With the growth of the training program in Austin and a very supportive medical community, the idea of a medical school was resurrected. In 2004 the Travis County Hospital District was created with funding provided by a voter referendum. Its stated goals was to provide health care through Brackenridge hospital to people below a specific level or poverty line. The hospital district evolved into what is now called Central Health. The ownership of Brackenridge Hospital was transferred to Central health in 2004. They also now manage the Medical Access Program (MAP) that provides payments for hospital services for the population of eligible residents who are at or below 100% of the federal poverty line. Central Health has also taken charge of multiple health care clinics formerly run by the City and County. One of the members of the Central Health board is Clarke Heidrick, who has been very active in civic affairs and has had much communication with the rest of the community. Dr. Tom Coopwood has also been active on the board of Central Health.

Subsequent to that notable development of creating a hospital district, several organizations became interested in this issue. The Austin Downtown Alliance, a partnership of business owners in the downtown area, felt that creating a medical school would be a very positive influence on improving the value and vitality of the center city. The Chamber of Commerce also became interested in the possibilities for enhancing business activities in the downtown area. In 2011, Senator Kirk Watson stated in his "10 in 10" goals speech on health care, that the creation of a Medical School would be one of those goals. With that kind of political support, along with much of the business community, the idea could move forward. The University of Texas at Austin had been interested for some years in the further development of biotechnology, engineering and bioscience in their departments on the campus.[80,81]

In 2012, the voters of Austin supported a tax increase that would maximize the receipt of new federal funds to be used in collaboration with Seton for health care. That included $35 million annually for a medical school. Seton and the Dell Foundation pledged funds for the creation of a medical school. The University of Texas Board of Regents pledged $25 million of annual funding to a UT Austin medical school plus $40 million over eight years for faculty recruiting. The State of Texas has provided $4.9 million to the Austin Community College for development of a biotechnology research and training facility where students would have access to training for jobs in that field. And the business community looks forward to the development of a number of innovative companies that may locate in the central east Austin area, near the medical school campus. This would fulfill the early concept of diversifying the economy for the future.

In January of 2014, Dr. S. Claiborne Johnston, was named the inaugural dean of the Dell Medical School. Dr. Sue Cox has been appointed the executive vice dean for academics. On June 29, 2015 the medical school was notified that it would receive preliminary accreditation that would allow it to start recruiting students. The initial class is expected to include fifty students. In 2015 the initial three buildings were started: the Health Learning Building, the primary learning area; the Health Discovery Building, primarily a research building; and the Health Transformation Building, which included doctors' offices, ambulatory surgery and demonstration clinics. In August of 2014, construction of the Dell Seton Medical Center at UT Hospital was begun. The Dell Medical School will not be a Health Science Center, but functions under the Dean of the University of Texas, Austin, unlike the other health science centers in Texas that report directly to the Chancellor of the UT system.

I look at this 85-year history of medical training as a tribute to a community with a remarkable group of doctors. This history involved a setting where a single intern came to a community hospital; was nurtured by a number of dedicated physicians; was the start of a long lasting program that evolved into a more organized system created by the medical society; and was further nourished by the contributions from distant resources at UTMB, UT Houston, St. Joseph Hospital and even collaborations with programs as far away Wyoming, New Mexico, Corpus Christi and San Antonio. As that has continued to grow, the training of a single trainee has morphed to a program involving over 250 residents and many more students. The efforts of a number of dedicated individuals have been multiplied into several hundred doctors and others to create a high-level community resource, including the University of Texas at Austin Dell Medical School.

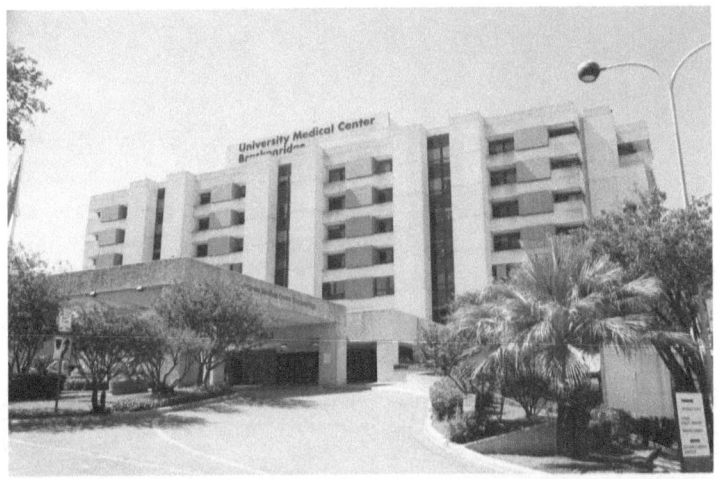

Brackenridge Hospital one week before all patients are moved out to the new Dell Seton Medical Center, May 13, 2017.

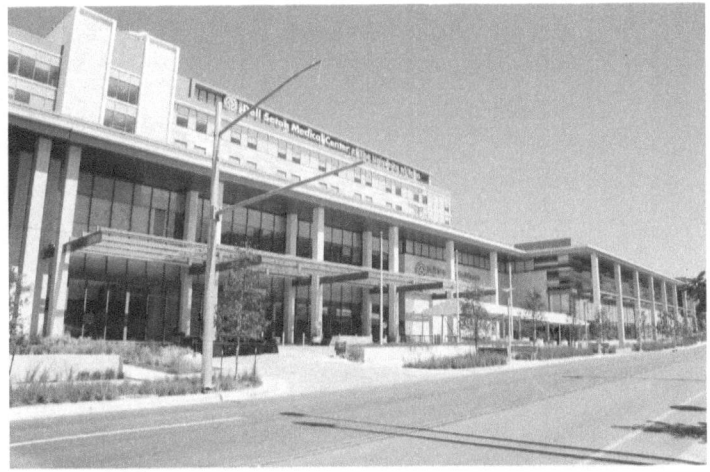

Dell Seton Medical Center at The University of Texas one week before patients are moved into the facility.

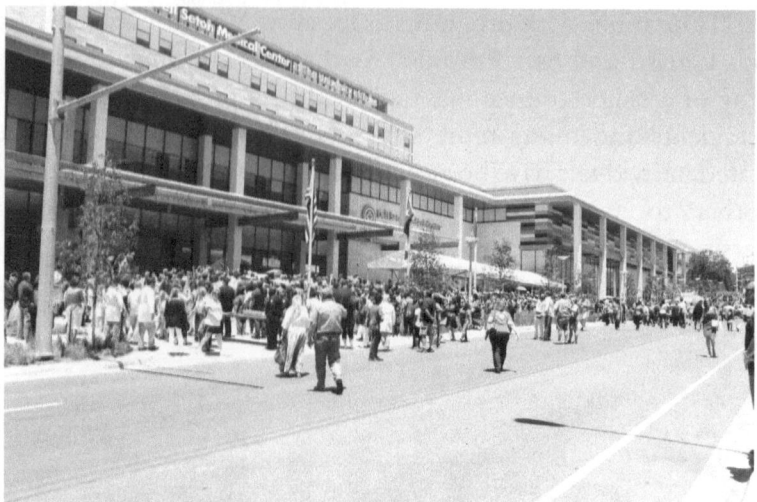

Dell Seton Medical Center with parade of people who walked form Brackenridge to celebrate the change from Brackenridge Hospital care to Dell Seton Medical Center care May 13, 2017.

Footnotes

1. The American Medical Association, Google search
2. U. S. Food and Drug Administration – Significant Dates FDA, http:// Google search
3. Lisa Fahrenthold, Sara Rider, "Admissions, the extraordinary History of Brackenridge Hospital" (Brackenridge Hospital, 1984)
4. "Stat News" Brackenridge Hospital Employee Publication, May 1969
5. Mary Mika, personal communication, 1998
6. Yale Journal of Medicine and Law: 'History of Medical Insurance in the United States" www.yalemmedlaw.com 2009
7. Mrs. Anita Land, RN -personal communication
8. Mrs. Jewel Fox, RN -personal communication
9. Joseph L.B DeLee, AM, MD "The Practical Medicine Series Obstetrics, Year Book Publishers 1929
10. J. Whilridge Williams, "Obstetrics", Sixth Edition, Appleton & Co. 1931
11. Arthur Hale Curtis, MD, "Obstetrics and Gynecology," Vol. II, W. B. Saunders Company 1933
12. "Stat News"
13. American Medical Association Archives.
14. Sam Wilburn, MD Obituary
15. Ruth M. Bain, MD with Marilyn Miller Baker, "Doors Will Open for You" Texas Women's University printing service, Denton Texas, 1997
16. "Texas Cousins" "Correll, Tisdale, and Related Families" Marie C. Tisdale and Albert A Tisdale, Nortex Press, Austin, Texas 1986
17. Kermit Fox, MD -personal communication
18. Georgia Legett -personal communications
19. Medical Staff Newsletter, Seton Family of Hospitals,Volume 26, issue 07, July 2007

20. Jane Lewis, -personal communication, Daughter of Dr. Bud Dryden
21. Dr. Clinton Cravens, MD -personal communication
22. Dr. Earl Grant, MD -personal connunication
23. "Remnisciences of a Texas Surgeon" R. Maurice Hood, MD, an autobiography 1994
24. Texas Department of State Health Services, "Texas Emergency Services History" dshs.texas.gov
25. Dickens v. United States. Civ.A. No. 72-H-1494. Leagle.com
26. Dr. Bob Pape, -personal communication
27. John Morthland, "St. David's, 90 Years and Counting" Texas Monthly Custom Publishing 2014
28. Mr. Bob Spurk -personal communication
29. Travis County Medial Society minutes, 1972
30. Dr. Bob Pape -personal communication
31. Keith Nobel, Austin EMS public relations officer, -personal communication
32. The National EMS Museum emsmuseum.org
33. Dr. Charles Felger -personal communication
34. Dr. John Boyd -personal communication
35. Dr. Norm Chenven -personal communication
36. Dr. Don Connel -personal communication
37. Dr. Al Lindsey -personal communication
38. Dr. Joun Blewett -personal communication
39. Dr. Ken Sherman -personal communication
40. Dr. Karen Teel -personal communication
41. Minutes Travis County Medical Society, March 1972
42. Dr. Tom Zavaleta -personal communication
43. Dr. George Edwards -personal communication
44. Dr. Richard Holt -personal communication
45. Dr. Jonathan Dechard -personal communication
46. Dr. Jack Schneider -personal communication
47. Dr. Earl Matthews -personal communication
48. Dr. Lysbeth Miller -personal communication
49. Dr. Clyde Smith -personal communication
50. Dr. Hector Morales -personal communication
51. Dr. David H. Harshaw -personal communication
52. Dr. Ben Coopwood -personal communication
53. Dr. Fred W. Hansen -personal communication
54. Dr. Terrance A Kuhlmann -personal communication
55. Dr. Eldrid Kaplan -personal communication

56. Dr. Gerald Mankovsky -personal communication
57. Dr. Richard Sjoberg -personal communication
58. Dr. Eric Upton -personal communication
59. Dr. Charles Brown -personal communication
60. Dr. Thomas Vaughn -personal communication
61. "Dr. Mathus Blackstock , An Austin Physician's Life" Document recorded by Dr. Jeanne Cook and Dr. Jacqueline Kerr based on interviews in 2011 and 2012.
62. Dr. Ruth Bain "Doors Will Open For You" (see #15)
63. Dr. John Smolik -personal communication
64. Dr. Terry Wiggins personal communication
65. Intern and residency listing from the training program office provided by Mary Mika
66. Dr. Mathus Blackstock "An Austin Physician's Life" Document recorded by Dr. Jeanne Cook and Dr. Jaqueline Kerr
67. Dr. David Wright -personal communication
68. Dr. Cynthia Brison -personal communication
69. Dr. Dana Sprute -personal communication
70. Dr. William Tierney -personal communication
71. Dr. Beverly J. Sutton -personal communication
72. Dr. Donald Parsons -personal communication
73. Dr. William J.Reitmeyer -personal communication
74. Dr. Suzanna Dana -personal communication
75. Dr. Phillip Collins -personal communication
76. Mr. Jack Campbell, former CEO of St. David's hospital -personal communication
77. Dr. James O. Lindsey -personal communication
78. Ascension Health -ascension.org
79. Dr. Sue Cox –personal communication
80. Mr. Clarke Heidrick -personal communication
81. Mr. Charles Betts –personal commuication
82. Mr. Marshall Cothran –personal communication

Appendix A

List of interns and residents 1931 to 2000
* doctors who stayed in Austin

George Bennack, M.D.	6/4/31-7/5/32
Claud Martin, M.D. *	6/32-7/33
Charles B. Dildy, M.D. *	1935
David. L. White, M.D.	1935-36
Tillman E. Dodd, M.D. *	1937
John T. Frawley, M.D.	1940
Sam W. Wilborn, M.D. *	1941
Ruth M. Bain, M.D. *	1942
Otto Brandt, Jr. M.D. *	1942
Wilbur Quinte Budd, M.D.	6/27/46-6/30/47
John H. Cayce, M.D.	4/1/47-5/1/48
Sigman W. Hayes, M.D. *	1948
Benjamin Elliott, M.D.	7/1/47-5/1/49
James W. Terrell, M.D.	1948-1949
James A. Walker, M.D.	1948-1949
Russell E. Youngberg, M.D.	1948-1949
James R. Sims Jr. M.D.	7/1/49-7/1/50

Interns 7/1/50-6/30/51
Richard C. Allen, Jr. M.D.
Robert E. Colbert, M.D.

Curtis B. Pillsbury, M.D.
John Haskell Tate, M.D.
John C. Wells, M.D.

Residents 1950-51

Charles E. Davis, M.D.	Medicine-Pediatrics 7/1/50-10/16/50 (military leave of absence)
Kenneth Reidland, M.D.	7/1/50-6/30/51 (Chief Surgery Resident)
Rafael S. Villareal, M.D.	7/1/50-12/31/50 Rotating 1/1/51-6/30/52 Med.-Peds.
Porfior Diaz, M.D.	1/1/51-6/30/52 Surgery

Interns 1951-1952
James W. Thomas, M.D. *
Frank R. Ervin, M.D.
Marvin H. Gohlke, M.D.
Henry B. Harvey, M.D.
Hollis A. Stafford, M.D.
Stanley E. Thompson, M.D,

Residents, second and third year
W. M. Gambrell, M.D.
Richard C. Allen, Jr. M.D.
Gudelia Padlan, M.D.
Curtice B. Pillsbury, M.D.
Rafael Villareal, M.D.

Interns 1952-53
Martin P. Leggett, M.D. *
Jerald R. Senter, M.D. *
John Dale Archer, M.D.
Hamilton W. Kilpatrick, III, M.D.

Interns 1953-54
Rollie E. Allen, M.D.

William H. Brown, M.D.
Ted Henderson Forsythe, M.D.   (Married chief OB nurse and they moved to Lubbock)

James E. Wilson, Jr. M.D.
Willard R. Karn, Jr., M.D.
Carl O. Ramzy, M.D.
Robert Lee Schoenvogel, M.D.
Richard E. Short, M.D.

Second and third Year Residents 1953-54
Henry Ward Bendel, M.D.   General Practice
Gerald E. Brandes, M.D.   General Practice
Benjamin Lacsamana, M.D. General Practice
Pura Santiago, M.D. Peds
Bernard L. Willett, M.D. Surgery
Frank J. Lee, M.D. OB-GYN

Interns and Residents 1954-55
Bill Ray Boring, M.D.   Tom E. Linstrum, M.D.
Sidney Richardson, M.D.   Travis Phelps, M.D.
James A. Fisher, M.D.   Robert s. Ray, M.D.
Buster E. McCoy, M.D.   Donald S. Kennady, M.D.
R. F. Sowell, M.D.   M. S. Madison, M.D.
William H. Andrew, Jr. M.D.   Donald M. Lowery, M.D.

Interns 1955-56
Billy Bob Alexander, M.D.   Norman Anderson, M.D.
Dan Bacon, M.D.   Charles Borchers, M.D.
Nobel Endicott, M.D.   Henry Allen Hooks, M.D
Richard Lane, M.D.   Frances Martin, M.D.
Lawrence Martin, M.D.   James Lloyd Spidle, M.D.*

OB Externs
Leroy Boriack, M.D.   Charles Hartel, M.D.
James Allison, M.D.   Charles Stevens, M.D.

OB-GYN Extern
Joseph Durso

Interns 1956-57
Capt. T. H. Barnett, M.D.
A. A. Bishop, M.D.
G. A Dawson, M.D.
Capt. Robert. P Rapp, M.D.*
Jack E. Tolar, M.D.
Larry H. Wharton, M.D.
Teddy M. Sousares, M.D.*

J. G. Barton, M.D.
D. A. Chester, M.D.
C. F. Campbell, M.D.
V. C. Smart, M.D. *
John J. Walker, M.D.
Robert W. Pape, M.D.*

OB-GYN Residents 1956-57
Charles Hartell, M.D.
L. M. Alvarez, M.D.
Robert Fahringer, M.D.

Interns 1957-58
Hulen J. Cook, M.D.
Charles E. Ford, M.D.
Donald H. Hopkins, M.D.
Thornton L. Kidd, Jr. M.D.
Francis E. McIntyre, M.D.*
Joseph S. Neight, M.D.
Charles L. Wolf, M.D.

Garland R. Dean, M.D.
Ralph G. Hodges, M.D.
Edward N. Jabalie, M.D.
Doran D. Maupin, M.D.
Richard McKee, M.D.
Lionel Rangel, M.D.

Residents OB-GYN 1957-58
Gaston Machado, M.D.
John Hutchison, M.D.

Interns 1958-59
Dan Spoor, M.D.
Hotchkiss, III, M.D.
William H Schiefelbein, M.D.
Jedd Green, M.D.
Angus Marshall, M.D.

Henry Moore, M.D.
James F. Eades, M.D.
Wagner, M.D.
William Nash, M.D.
Max C. Butler, M.D.

George A. Gant, M.D.
Earl F. Grant, M.D.*
Cecil L. Henkel, M.D.
Bobby Joe Smith, M.D.*

Resident, Surgery 1958-59
Leonard Coleman, M.D.

Interns 1959-60
W. S. Smith, M.D.
Charles Primer, M.D.
Leroy Schaffnr, M.D.
D. A. Baggett, M.D. *
Jack Tolar, M.D.
Joyce Wilson, M.D.
W. D. Bailey, M.D.
Abe G. Rodriguez, M.D. *

Interns 1960-61
Ann T. Bouldin, M.D.
Robert R. Burns, M.D.
Billy M. Dickey, M.D.
William D. King, M.D.
Charles G. Plyler, M.D.
Milton J. Railey, M.D.*
William R. Womack, Jr., M.D.
Vann A. Brewester, M.D.
Jerry H. Damon, M.D.
Orland D. Eliason, M.D.
Allen K. Heacock, M.D.
Craig Poindexter, M.D.
William Risk, M.D.

Residents 1960-61
Anthony N. Manoli, M.D. 2nd year
Norman Anderson Jr. M.D. 3rd year
Robert W. Pape, M.D. 1st year surgery*
Leroy Schaffner, M.D.

Interns 1961-62
Charles F. Butler, M.D.
Forrest Eisnerich, M.D.
Betty McElroy, M.D.
Marvin C. Overton, M.D.
Pat M. Tolar, M.D.
Jimme R. Clemons, M.D. *
Julius Kramer, M.D.*
Ross A. McElroy, M.D.
Lloyd Thompson, M.D.

Residents 1961-62
William Risk, M.D. 1st year
Robert W. Pape, M.D., 2nd year Surgery
Anthony N. Manoli, M.D. 3rd years

Interns 1962-63
L. E. Arnold, M.D. *
Fred B. Anderson, M.D.
Leslie r. Bornfleth, M.D.
Clinton E. Craven, M.D. *
John L. Humphrey, M.D.
Robert A. Tate, M.D. *
Harvey M. Williams, M.D.

Robert S. Alexander, M.D.
Henry J. Boehm, M.D.
Glenn C. Coates, M.D.
Houston. G. Hambry, M.D.
Gary N. Pamplin, M.D.*
Willis M. Thorstad, M.D. *

Residents 1962-63
J. Fred Kramer, M.D. 1st year Surgery
Robert W. Pape, M.D. 2nd year surgery

Interns 1963-64
James R. Finch, M.D.
William L. Lemon, M.D.
June E. Richardson, M.D. *

Capt. Gary R. Jones, M.D. *
Edwin E. Owens, M.D.

Residents 1963-64
Waldo A. Gonzalez, M.D. 1st year surgery
Milton H. Stern. M.D.
Capt. Lawrence J. Stuart, M.D.
Herman R. Van Sickle, M.D.
James Thomas Walker, M.D.

Interns 1964-65
Dana B. Copp, M.D.
Fredrick F. Petmecky, M.D.
Presley Joe Mock, Jr., M.D.

Walter r. Konzen, M.D.
Charles E. Strauss, M.D.
Richard L. Ballard, M.D.*

Residents 1964-65
J. Fred Kramer, M.D. (Chief Surgical Resident)
Franklin C. Harmon, M.D. (Surgery)
James L. Spidle, M.D. (Pathology, 1st year)*
Norman Miles, M.D. (OB-GYN)
David Haggard, M.D. (OB-GYN)

Interns 1965-66

Travis L. Casler, M.D.
Robert Davis, M.D.
Vernon E. Grove, M.D.*
Richard Orr. M.D.
Joe R. Reneau, M.D.*
Richard L. Weddige, M.D.

Howard B. Condren, M.D.
Ralph H. Gay, M.D.
Robert Hazlewood, M.D. *
Robert Potts, M.D.
Samuel H. Shaddock, M.D.

Residents 1965-66
F. C. Harmon Jr. (Chief resident Surgery)
Robert A. Tate, M.D. (1st year Surgery)*
James A. Spidle, M.D. (2nd year Pathology)*
Sidney Smith, M.D. (OB-Gyn)
Michael Howard, M.D. (OB-GYN)
James Taylor Wharton, M.D. (OB-GYN)

Interns 1966-67

Weldon L. Ash, M.D.
Everett Martin Donowho, M.D.
Curtis S. Heinrich, M.D.
Thomas F. Lowe, M.D.
Lynn R. Nesbitt, M.D.

Michael J. Doughety, M.D.
Thomas P. Fagan, M.D.
F. Howard Hughes, M.D.
Charles M. Myers, M.D.
R. Al Trompler, M.D.

Residents 1966-67
Robert A. Tate, M.D. (2nd year Surgery)*
James A. Spidle, M.D. (3rd year Pathology)*
Francisco Veloz, M.D. (1st year Surgery)
Pramool Sukawatana, M.D.

Interns 1967-68
John Baker, M.D.*
Han Howard, M.D.
Bill Schuesler, M.D.
James Winn, M.D.

Raymond Buck, M.D.
Dicky Huey, M.D.
Alfred Wiliams, M.D.

Residents 1967-68
Robert A. Tate, M.D. (3rd year Surgery)*
Ricky Donowho, M.D. (1st year)
James Spidle, M.D. (4th year Pathology)*
Francisco Veloz, M.D. (2nd year Surgery)
David Shannon, M.D.
Pedro Guiroga, M.D.

Travis Casler, M.D.

Gene Jones, M.D.

Interns 1968-69
Kenneth O. Albers, M.D.
O. Preston Copeland, M.D.
Harry A. Croft, M.D.
Daniel M. Kelly, M.D.
Charles L. Mott, M.D.*
Bruno Anderson, M.D.

Bruce M. Bauknight, M.D.
John A Craig. M.D. *
Phillip M. Kassner, M.D.
Janusz A. Konikowski, MD
Bert B. Oubre, M.D.
Oscar Sotelo, M.D.

Interns 1969-70
Fred Ames, M.D.
Bill Bass, M.D.
Don Howard, M.D.
Fay Mott, M.D.
Hayne Sheffield, M.D.

Tarfer Bailey, M.D.
Charles Hill, M.D.
Jim McNabb, M.D. *
Stan Novy, M.D.
Mike Stewart, M.D.

Residents 1969-70
Paulo F. L. Becker, M.D. (2nd year Pathology)
Ray Buck, M.D. (2nd year Surgery)
Pierre Greef, M.D. (2nd year Surgery)
Ken Fannin, M.D. (Chief Resident, Surgery)*

Interns 1970-71

Jack Bankhead, M.D.
Thomas Blucker, M.D.
Can Cravy, M.D.
Bobby Maddox, M.D.

John Bannister, M.D.
Sharon Bowen, M.D.
William Jones, M.D. *

Residents 1970-71

Ray Buck, M.D. (3rd year Surgery)
Mary Mauldin, M.D.
Joun Price, M.D.
Ken Teufel, M.D.
Thomas Wascher, M.D.
William T. Miller, M.D.

Boonlau Yardee, M.D.
William Peterek, M.D.
Paul Redman, M.D.
Rodney Traeger, M.D.
Peter De. Ipolyi, M.D.
Halsey M. Settle, III, M.D.

Interns 1971-72

Robert O. Collier, M.D.
Richard T. Herrick, M.D.
Thomas J. Lawhon, M.D.
John D. Oswalt, M.D. *
Thomas M. Smith, M.D.
Travis L. Warthan, M.D.
Milton C. Wlliams, M.D.

Larry R. Delane, M.D.
Philip T. Labarbera, M.D.
Thomas B. McIntosh, M.D.
B. B. Prestridge, M.D.
David K. Teegarden, M.D.
Hugh N. West, M.D.

Interns 1972-73

John R. Boyd, M.D. *
Dennis M. Lanier, M.D.
Harvey Renger, M.D. *
Wade H. Smith, M.D.
Robert R. Wallis, M.D.

Henry C. Harper, M.D.
Robert C. Northcutt, M.D.
Terry J. Sherman, M.D. *
Joe P. Treadaway, M.D.

Interns 1973-74

William Bucholtz, M.D. (withdrew 7/30/73)
Constance Hanna, M.D. *
Hardy Morgan, M.D.

Jary Morgan, M.D.
Wilmer Lynn Reep, M.D. George B. Talley, M.D.

Resident 1973-74
Charles D. Bell, M.D. (10/1/73- 9/30/74)

The start of CTMF. (End of free-standing rotating internships.) Some are "Flexible Interns" 1974-75

Royal B. Anspach, M.D.
Ira Bell, M.D. (Starts rotating intern, joins family practice)*
Jonathan Chancellor, M.D.   James Eggers, M.D.
Gerald W. Growcock, M.D.   David J Jacoby, M.D.
Jack W. Janoe, M.D.   Hans A. Langsjoen, M.D.
Sidney T. Robin, M.D. *   Robert C. Schwartz, M.D.
Terry S. Wiggins. M.D. * (joins family practice residency)
Douglas W. Wohlfahrt, M.D.* (Joins family practice residency)
Philip L. Zbylot, M.D.

Flexible Interns 1975-76
John Birsner, M.D.   Bruce Cox, M.D.
Lance LeDoux, M.D.   D. S. Reddy, M.D.
Clyde Rutherford, M.D.

Family Practice Residents 1975-76

First Year
Abraham Delgsdo, M.D.   Louis Hill, M.D.
E. John Smolik, M.D.*   Lynn Warthan, M.D.*
Second Year
Ira Bell, M.D. *   Terry Wiggins, M.D. *
Douglas Wohlfahrt, M.D. *
Third Year
Connie Hanna, M.D. *   Hardy Morgan, M.D.

Internal Medicine 1975-76

Interns
Richard Johnston, M.D.
Richard Marietta, M.D.
Charles Moore, M.D. *

Bob Dodd, M.D.
Nelson Vicuna, M.D.

First Year Residents
Roger Aertker, M.D.
Nao-Hsiung Hung, M.D.
Michael Maros, M.D.

Robert Schwartz, M.D.
Carlos E. Zamora, M.D.

Second Year Residents
Lowell Chaffin, M.D.
Thomas Guerra, M.D.

Ken Smith, M.D.
Dan Finch, M.D. *

Third year Residents
Pete Ethridge, M.D.

Pathology residents

1st year Residents
Paul LeBourgouis, M.D.
William Reitmeyer, M.D. *

4th year Residents
Charles Bell, M.D.

Pediatric Residents 1975-76

1st year Residents
Charlotte Ann Weaver, M.D. *
Robin Mers, M.D.

Michael Green, M.D.

2nd year Residents
Najma Khan, M.D.
Tom Zavaleta, M.D. *

Michael Bryne, M.D.

3rd year Residents
Terry Furguiele, M.D.

HOUSE STAFF, CTMF 1976-77

Flexible Interns
Theresa Brevard, M.D.

John Durfor, M.D.

Muneera Hahood, M.D.
David Sawyer, M.D.
Wes Wallace, M.D.

Charles Sadler, M.D.
Frank Stagg, M.D.

Family Practice Residents
1st years
Joan Frazier, M.D.
Robert Millikan, M.D.
Kenneth B Swerman, M.D.

Joseph Malleske, M.D.
Robert Youens, M.D.

2nd year
Louis Hill, M.D.

3rd year
Ira Bell, M.D.*
Douglas Wohlfahrt, M.D. *

Terry Wiggins, M.D. *
Lynn Warthan, M.D. *

Internal Medicine
Interns
John Nelson, M.D.
Paula Noelke, M.D.
Robert Griffin, M.D. *

Patricia Rush, M.D.
Mark Werner, M.D.

1st year
Richard Johnston. M.D.
Charles Moore, M.D. *
Clyde Lee Rutherford, M.D.

Richard Marietta, M.D.
Bob Dodd, M.D.

2nd year
Roger Aertker, M.D.
Michael Maros, M.D.

Mao-Hsiung Hung, M.D.
Carlos E. Zamora, M.D.

3rd year
Tom Guerra, M.D.
Dan Finch, M.D. *

Ken Smith, M.D.

Pathology Residents 2nd year
Paul Lebougouis, M.D.
William Reitmeyer, M.D *

Pediatric Residents

1st year
Martha Steele, M.D.
Tim Mangan, M.D.

Ralph DuBose, M.D.
Jim Garner, M.D.

2nd year
Charlotte Ann Weaver, M.D.*
Robin Mers, M.D.

Michael Green, M.D.
Sandy Adelman, M.D.

3rd year
Tom Zavaleta, M.D.*

HOUSE STAFF, CTMF 1977-78

Flexible Interns
Deborah Brown, M.D.
Christopher Chitambar, M.D.
John Rowe, M.D.

Louis Dickey, M.D.
Kent Roberts, M.D.
Marilyn Vache, M.D.

Family Practice

1st year
Mario Pena, M.D.
Clark Race, M.D.*
Clarence Porter, M.D.

Katherine Perkins, M.D.
George Smith, M.D.

2nd year
Joseph Malleske, M.D.
Robert Youens, M.D.
Pablo Garza, M.D.

Robert Millikan, M.D.
Peter Takhar, M.D.

3rd year
Louis R. Hill, M.D.

Pediatrics

1st year
Richard Beauchamps, M.D.
David (Randy) Ralph, M.D.

Theresa Brevard, M.D.
Forooz Mirza, M.D.

2nd year
Martha Steele, M.D.

Tim Mangan, M.D.

Jim Garner, M.D.
3rd year
Charlotte Ann Weaver, M.D.*
Sandy Adelman, M.D.

H. S. Chana, M.D.

Robin Mers. M.D.

Internal Medicine
Interns
Carolyn Oliver, M.D.
Laura Johnson Guerrero. M.D.
Archie Dan Smith, M.D. *
1st year
Paula Noelke, M.D.
Patricia Rush, M.D
2nd year
Richard Johnston, M.D.
Charles Moore, M.D. *
Clyde Lee Rutherford, M.D.
3rd year
Roger Aertker, M.D.*
Carlos E. Zamora, M.D.

John Marietta, M.D.*
Sarah Minden, M.D.

Robert Griffin. M.D.*
Mark Werner, M.D.

Richard Marietta, M.D.
Bob Dodd, M.D.

Michael Maros, M.D.

Pathology Residents
Paul LeBourgouis, M.D.
William Reitmeyer, M.D.8

HOUSE STAFF 1978-1979

Flexible Interns
David Greene, M.D.
Will Chickering, MD.

Doreen Mowers, M.D.
James Sauer, M.D.

Family Medicine
1st year
Thomas Hayes, M.D.
Russell Krienke, M.D.

Amy Jones, M.D.
Alfonso Ramirez, M.D.

Doug Rankin, M.D.
2nd year
Katherine Perkins, M. D.
Clarence Porter, M. D.
Harold Woodward, M.D.
3rd year
Bobby Youens, M.D.
Joe Malleske, M.D.
Pablo Garza, M.D.

Sam Roberts, M.D.

Clark Race, M. D.
George Smith, M.D.

Randy Millikan M, D.
Perer Takhar, M.D.

Internal Medicine
Interns
Michael McElveen, M.D.
Wade Peters, M. D.
Ed Garcia, M.D.
1st year
Abe Delgado, M.D.
Laura Guerrero, M.D.
A. D. Smith, M.D.
2nd year
Paula Noelke, M.D.
Mark Werner, M.D.

Tom Hoffman, M.D.
Scott Gremillion, M. D.

Chirs Chitambar, M.D.
John Marietta, M.D.

Robert Griffin, M.D.

Nephrology Fellow
Clyde Lee Rutherford, M.D.

Pediatrics
1st year
Charles Michael Rios, M.D.
2nd year
Richard Beauchamp, M.D.
Randy Ralph, M.D.
3rd year
Marty Steele, M.D.
Jim Garner, M. D.

Antonio Calderon, M.D.

Theresa Breevard, M.D.
Forooq Mirza, M. D.

Tim Mangan, M.D.
H. S. Chana, M.D.

HOUSE STAFF 1979-1980

Flexible Interns
Jane Monts, M.D.
Charles Fazio, M.D.
Bonnie Stump, M.D.

Geoff Glidden, M.D.
Richard Yee, M.D.

Family Practice
1st year
Robert Howard, M.D.
Mark Wilson, M.D.
Patsy Jones, M.D.
2nd year
Thomas Hayes, M.D.
Doug Rankin, M.D.
Will Chickering, M.D.
3rd year
Katherine Perkins M.D
Clarence Porter, M.D.
Peter Takhar, M.D.

Ann Trentin, M.D.
Randy Reid, M.D.
Austin Weaver, M.D.

Russell Krienke, M.D.
Sam Roberts, M.D.
Alfonzo Ramirez, M.D.

Jim Hartye, M.D.
George Smith, M.D.

Internal Medicine
1st year
Leslie Cortes, M.D.
Marc Schatte, M.D.
2nd year
Mario Juarez, M.D.
Scott Gremillion, M.D.
3rd year
Chris Chitambar, M.D.
Laura Guerrero, M.D.
A. D. Smith, M.D.
4th year
Bob Griffin, M.D.

Tom Marker, M.D.
Michael Smith, M.D.

Nap Mayorga, M.D.
Eddie Garcia, M.D.

Abe Delgado, M.D.
John Marietta, M.D.

Pediatrics
1st year
Peggy Abel, M.D.
Larry Smith, M.D.
2nd year
Lily Sood, M.D.
Farooq Mirza, M.D.
3rd year
Richard Beauchamp, M.D.

Don Sartor, M. D.
Karen Codjoe, M.D.

Mike Rios, M.D.

Nephrology Fellow
Lee Rutherford, M.D.

John Nelson, M.D.

Pathology
Randy Ralph, M.D.

Surgery
Phil Lindsay, M.D.
William Powell, M.D.

Valerie Wright, M.D.
Robert Wright, M.D.

HOUSE STAFF 1980-1981

Flexible Interns
Rob Reeb, M.D.
Leigh Fincher, M.D.
George Martinez, M.D.

Gayl Gustafson, M.D.
David Ugland, M.D.
Paul Subart, M.D.

Family Practice
1st year
John Berman, M.D.
Michael Dennis, M.D.
Peggy Russell, D.O.
2nd year
Robert Howard, M.D.
Mark Wilson, M.D.

Kenneth Blair, M.D,
Dirk Havlak, M.D.
David Wright, M.D.

Ann Trentin, M.D.
Randy Reid, M.D.

Patsy Jones, M.D.
3rd year
Russell Krienke, M.D.
Sam Roberts, M.D.
Alfonso Ramirez, M.D.

Austin Weaver, M.D.

Doug Rankin, M.D.
Will Chickering, M.D.

Pediatrics
1st year
A. Raof El-Din, M.D
Peggy Abel, M.D.
Alfa Bornate-Garcia, M.D.
2nd year
Don Sartor, M.D.
Nena Piga, M.D.
3rd year
Lily Sood, M.D.
Farooq Mirza, M.D.

Bernadette Brown, M.D.
Patrick Dwyer, M.D.
Susan Panfield, M.D.

Karen Codjoe, M.D.

Kike Rios, M.D.

Internal Medicine
1st year
Ricardo Alvillar, M.D.
Linda Dooley, M.D.
Cass Ragan, M.D.
2nd year
Steve Wilkening, M.D.
Tom Marker, M.D.
Joseph Cotrepia, M.D.
3rd year
Nap Mayorga, M.D.
Eddie Garcia, M.D.
4th year
A. D. Smith, M.D.

John Bagwell, M.D.
Tom MacDermaid, M.D.

Leslie Cortes, M.D.
Michael Smith, M.D.

Scott Gremillion, M.D.
Abe Delgado, M.D.

Pathology
2nd year
Randy Ralph, M.D.

Suzanna Dana, M.D.

HOUSE STAFF 1981-1982

Flexible Interns
John Connolly, M.D.
John Frodel, M.D.
Chip Klunick, M.D.

Mark Crozier, M.D.
Tom Kittleman, M.D.
Stephen Marin, M.D.

Family Practice
1st year
James Bartay, M.D.
Barrett Hays, M.D.
Carla Underhill, M.D.

Gary Beach, M.D.
David Pampe, M.D.
Mary Uptam, M.D.

2nd year
John Berman, M.D.
Michael Dennis, M.D.
David Wright, M.D.

Kennith Blair, M.D.
Dirk Havlak, M.D.
George Martinez, M.D.

3rd years
Robert Howard, M.D.
Mark Wilson, M.D.
Patsy Jones, M.D.

Ann Trentin, M.D.
Randy Reid, M.D.
Austin Weaver, M.D.

Pediatrics
1st year
Valerie Beckles, M.D.
Harpreet Grewal, M.D.

Shyamala Johnson, M.D.
Reyner Ildefonzo, M.D.

2nd year
Bernadette Brown, M.D.
Pat Dwyer, M.D.

Peggy Abel, M.D.
Susan Penfield, M.D.

3rd year
Don Sartor, M.D.
Nina Piga, M.D.

Maren Codjoe, M.D.
Lily Sood, M.D.

4th year
Mike Rios

Internal Medicine
1st year
David Dominguez, M.D. Bob Bret, M.D.
Steve Parker, M.D. Marsha Staats, M.D.
Jeanne Wham, M.D.
2nd year
Peggy Russell, D.O. Richardo Alvillar, M.D.
Linda Dooley, M.D. Tom MacDermaid, M.D.
Joseph Cotropia, M.D.
3rd year
Steve Wilkening, M.D. Leslie Cortes, M.D.
Tom Marker, M.D. Michael Smith, M.D.
Jere Robinson, M.D.

Patology
2nd year
Suzana Dana, M.D. Randy Ralph, M.D.

HOUSE STAFF 1982-1983

Flexible Interns
James R. Brown, M.D. John Flanagan, M.D.
James F. Hefner, M.D. R. Kim Keeland, M.D.
Cynthis Jeanne Lee, M.D. Richard W. Redfern, M.D.

Family Practice
PL-1
Ruben Aleman, M.D. John A. Calomeni, M.D.
Mark c. Dawaon, M.D. Eileen K. Hammar, M.D.
Robert Norris, M.D. Eward P Tyson, M.D.
PL-2
James Bartay, M.D. Gary Beach, M.D.
Barrett Hays, M.D. David Pampe, M.D.
Carla Underhill, M.D. Kathy Upham, M.D.
PL-3
John Berman, M.D. Kenneth Blair, M.D.

Michael Dennis, M.D
David Wright, M.D.

Dirk Havlak, M.D.
George Martinez, M.D.

Internal Medicine
PL-1
Don P. Bunnell, M.D.
Alton Graham, M.D.
Rosalind F. Hudson. M.D.
PL-2
Dominguez, M.D.
Steve Parker, M.D.
Jeanne Wham, M.D.
PL-3
Peggy Russell, D.O
Linda Dooley, M.D.
Joseph Cotropia, M.D.

James D. Colson, M.D.
Pamela J. Hendrickson, M.D.

Bob Bret, M.D.
Marsha Staats, M.D.

Ricardo Alvillar, M.D.
Tom MacDermaid, M.D.

Pediatrics
PL-1
Casey Mulcihy, M.D.
Tahira Malek, M.D.
Herleen Kailey, M.D.
PL-2
Antonio Loiz, M.D.
PL-3
Pat Dwyer, M.D.
Susan Penfield, M.D.

Mrudula Deshpande, M.D.
John Harmon, M.D.
Samara Turner, M.D.

Valerie Beckles, M.D.

Bernadette Brown, M.D.
Rudy Barrera, M.D.

Pathology
1PL-1
Robert S. Zirl, M.D.
Pl-4
Suzanna Dana, M.D.

Robert S. Hanes. M.D.

HOUSE STAFF 1983-1984

Flexible Interns
DonWillis, M.D.
Jim Pickens, M.D.
Harry Rosenthal, M.D.
Elizabeth Cissy Kraft, M.D.
Gail Hovorka, M.D.
John Liu, M.D.

Family Practice
PL-1
Gwendolyn Allen, M.D.
James Holloy, M.D.
Dan Ramsey, M.D.
Larry Baros, M.D.
Thomas Raetzch, M.D.
Edward Reed, M.D.
PL-2
Ruben Aleman, M.D.
Robert Norris, M.D.
Jim Brown, M.D.
Mark Dawson, M.D.
Edward Tyson, M.D.
C. Jeanne Lee, M.D.
PL-3
James Bartay, M.D.
Barrett Hays, M.D.
Carla Underhill, M.D.
Gary Beach, M.D.
David Pampe, M.D.
Kathy Upham, M.D.

Internal Medicine
PL-1
Brent Coleman, D.O.
Tom Hunt, M.D.
Doug Mills, M.D.
Tony Hannaman, M.D.
Hugh Mewhinney, M.D.
PL-2
Alton Graham, M.D.
Rosalind Hudson, M.D.
Margaret Clark. M.D.
Pam Hendrickson, M.D.
Diana Wallace, M.D.
PL-3
David Dominguez, M.D.
Steve Parker, M.D.
Jeanne Wham. M.D.
Bob Bret, M.D.
Marsha Staats, M.D.

PL-4
Peggy Russell, D.O.

Pediatrics
L-1
Cheryl Coldwater, M.D.
Maria Antigua, M.D.
PL-2
Marielou Guzon, M.D.
Drudula Deshande, M.D.
Herleen Kailey, M.D.
PL-3
Antonia Loiz, M.D.

Khodayar Rais-Bahrami, M.D.
Ernesto Ferrer, M.D.

Casey Mulcihy, M.D.
Tahira Malik, M.D.
Samara Turner, M.D.

Valerie Beckles, M.D.

Pathology
PL-1
Cory Jammal, M.D.
PL-2
Robert S. Zirl, M.D.

Robert S. Hanes, M.D.

HOUSE STAFF 1984-1985

Flexible Interns
Art Boone M.D.
Graves Hearnsberger, M.D.
Mike McIntyre, M.D.

Joel Carp, M.D.
Terry Jones, M.D.
Alan Rogers, M.D.

Family Practice
PL-1
Ann Bartolotta, M.D.
Georia Milan, M.D.
Dora Salazar, M.D.
PL-2
Larry Baros, M.D.
Cissy Craft, M.D.

Paul Bristol, M.D.
Gary Piefer, M.D.
john Weaver, M.D.

Lames Molloy, M.D.
Thomas Raetzch, M.D.

Dan Ramsey, M.D.
PL-3
Ruben Aleman, M.D.
Robert Norris, M.D.
Jim Brown, M.D.

Edward Reed, M.D.

Mark Dawson, M.D.
Edward Tyson, M.D.
C. Jeanne Lee, M.D.

Internal Medicine
PL-1
David Greene, M.D.
Ellen Remenchik, M.D.
Winton Watkins, M.D.
PL-2
Carlos Herrera, M.D.
Tony Hannaman, M.D.
Doug Mills, M.D.
PL-3
Alton Graham, M.D.
Rosalind Hudson, M.D.
Alice Penrose, M.D.
PL-4
Jeanne Wham, M.D.

Ed Lewis, M.D.
Scott Spoor, M.D.

Brent Coleman, M.D.
Tom Hunt, M.D.

Pam Hendrickson, M.D.
Margaret Clark, M.D.

Pediatrics
PL-1
Alice Seaton, M.D.
Mary Parks, M.D.
Minaxi Parekh, M.D.
PL-2
Cheryl Coldwater, M.D.
Maria Antigua, M.D.
PL-3
Marielou Guzon, M.D.
Mrudula Deshpande, M.D.
Herleen Kailey, M.D.

Enrique Quintero, M.D.
David Halioo, M.D.

Khodayar Rais-Bahrami, M.D.
Ernesto Ferrer, M.D.

Casey Mulcihy, M.D.
Tahira Malik M.D.
Samara Turner, M.D.

Pathology
PL-1
Randy Eckert, M.D.

HOUSE STAFF 1985-1986

Flexible Interns
Richard M. Bond, M.D.
Jay M. Rubin, M.D.
Rex P. Spear, M.D.
John D. O'Neil, M.D.
Barry S. Seibel, M.D.
Gregory P. Swanson, M.D.

Family Practice
PL-1
Sylvia A. Proctor Adams, M.D.
George L. Kneller, M.D.
Lorraine K. Schroeder. M.D.
Gwendolyn Allen. M.D.
Carmen C. Purl, M.D.
Eric W. Weidmann, M.D.
PL-2
Ann P. Bartolotta, M.D.
Georgia A. Milan, M.D.
Dora L. Salazar, M.D.
Paul E. Bristol. M.D.
Gary W. Piefer, M.D.
John D. Weaver, M.D.
PL-3
Larry W. Baros, M.D.
James P. Molloy, M.D.
Daniel E. Ramsey, M.D.
Elizabeth S. Kraft, M.D.
Thomas H. Raetzch, M.D.
Edward M. Reed, M.D.

Internal Medicine
PL-1
Stewart C. Birse, M.D.
Christine T. Malone, M.D.
Claudia S. Miller. M.D.
Kenneth C. Kroll, M.D.
Mary S. Maxwell, M.D.
PL-2
Arthur R. Boone, M.D.
Ellen M. Remenchek, M.D.
Winston E. Watkins, M.D.
David A. Greene, M.D.
Scott D. Spoor, M.D.

PL-3
Brent J Coleman, D.O.
Carlos, R. Herrera, M.D.

Robert A. Hannaman, M.D.
Thomas L. Hunt, M.D.

Pamela J. Hendrickson, M.D. Chief Resident to Dec. 1985
R. Douglas Mills, M.D. Chief resident 1/1/86-6/30/86

Pediatrics
PL-1
Ruth E. Archer. M.D.
Eufrosina A. T Lua, M.D.
Robert W. Wieting III, M.D.

Ezam Ghodsi, M.D.
Jayashree Mani, M.D.

PL-2
Manaxi P. Parekh, M.D.
Enrique T. Quintero, M.D.

Mary L. Park, M.D.
Alice M. Seaton, M.D.

PL-3
Maria B. Antigua, M.D.
Ernesto Ferrer, M.D.
Khodayar Rais-Bahrami, M.D.

Cheryl L. Coldwater, M.D.
Hou-The Lu, M.D.

Pathology
E. Randy Eckert

HOUSE STAFF 1986-1987

Transitional Interns
John W. Day, M.D.
Charlotte F. Hoehne, M.D
Juaquin Martiez, III, M.D.

Rebecca J. Driskell, M.D.
Charles M. Kasbarian, M.D.
Barry D. Meyer, M.D.

Family Practice
PL-1
Jeanne W. Cook, M.D.
Jacqueline M. Kerr, M.D.
Wail Malaty, M.D.

Philip Pe-Wen Huang, M.D.
Walter R. Leverich. M.D.
Rebecca A. McDonald, M.D.

PL-2
Sylvia A. Proctor-Adams, M.D.
George L. Kneller, M.D.
Larraine K. Schroeder, M.D.
PL-3
Ann B Bartolotta, M.D.
George A. Milan, M.D.
Dora L. Salazar, M.D.

Gwendolyn Allen, M.D.
Carmen C Purl, M.D.
Eric W. Weidmann, M.D.

Paul E. Bristol. M.D.
Gary W. Piefer, M.D.
John D. Weaver, M.D.

Internal Medicine
PL-1
Guy R. Gullion II, M.D.
Robert G. Huth, M.D.
Darrell E. Wilburn, M.D.
PL-2
Stewart C. Birse, M.D.
Christine T. Malone, M.D.
Claudia s. Miller, M.D.
PL-3
Arthur R. Boone, M.D.
Ellen J. Remenchek, M.D.

William L. Heeth, M.D.
Mark A. Prange, M.D.

Kenneth C Croll, M.D.
Mary S. Maxwell, M.D.

David A. Greene, M.D.
Scott D. Spoor, M.D. (Chief 1/1-6/1/87
Winston E. Watkins, M.D.

Carlos R. Herrera, M.D. (Chief Resident 7/1/86-12/31/86

Pediatrics
PL-1
Ricardo E. Calvo, M.D.
Donald K. Murphey, M.D.
Joanna K. Ramseyer-Weinberg, M.D.
PL-2
Ruth E. Archer, M.D.
Eufrosina A. Y. Lua, M.D.
Monica L. Suchoff, M.D.

Lee N. Muecke, M.D.
Eduardo A. Otero, M.D.

Ezam Ghodsi, M.D.
Jayashree Mani, M.D.
Robert W. Wieting, III, M.D.

PL-3
Manaxi P. Parekh, M.D.
Enrique T. Quintero, M.D.
Maria B. Antigua, M.D. (Chief Resident 7/1/86-12/31/86)

Mary P. Park, M.D.
Alice M. Seaton, M.D.

Pathology
PL-3
Edward R. Eckert, M.D. to 12/31/86

General Surgery
PL-3
Elizabeth T. Bonefas, M.D.
Gary Kubalak, M.D.
PL-4
Jean-Pierre Forage, M.D.
Michael Cosselli, M.D.
PL-5
Arthur Helllman, M.D.
T. O. Pouw, M.D.

Daniel Casse, M.D.
Dennis Meurer, M.D.

Phillip w. Jones, M.D.

E. L. Etter, II, M.D.

HOUSE STAFF 1987- 1988

Transitional Interns
Sandra S. Hatch, M.D.
Cullen A. McAllen, M.D.
John R. Taylor, M.D.

Charles A. Johnson, M.D.
John C. Smith, M.D.
Jon A. Yokubaitis, M.D.

Family Practice
PL-1
Carol M Byler, M.D.
Lisa B. Glenn, M.D.
David G. Joseph, M.D.
PL-2
Sylvia A. Adams, M.D.

Baldemar Covarrubial, M. D.
Horace G. Hinson, M.D.
Paul D. Keinarth, M.D.

Jeanne W. Cook, M.D.

Rebecca A. de la Torre, M.D.
Jacqueline M. Kerr, M.D.
Wail Malaty, M.D.
PL-3
Gwendolyn Allen, M.D.
Georgia A. Milan, M.D.
Lorraine K. Schroeder, M.D.
(Resident 7/1/87-6/30/88)

Philip P Huang, M.D.
Walter R. Leverich, M.D.

George L. Kneller, M.D.
Carmen C Purl, M.D.
Eric W. Weidmann, M.D.

Internal Medicine
PL-1
Rebecca Ellison, M.D.
Matthew E. Masters, M.D.
Terri T. Steele, M.D.
PL-2
Maria r. Gallego, M.D.
Robert G. Huth, M.D.
Darrell e. Wilburn, M.D.
PL-3
Stewart B. Birse, M.D.
Chief Res. 1/1-6/30/88
Christine T. Malone, M.D.
Claudia s. Miller M.D.
Chief Res. 7/1012/31/87

Carol Friedman, D.O.
Alina M. Ramos, M.D.

Barbara Fedor, M.D.
Mark A. Prange, M.D.

Kenneth C. Kroll, M.D.

Mary S. Maxwell, M.D.
Arthur R. Boone, M.D

Pediatrics
PL-1
Alena Ashenberg, M.D.
Truett a. Hull, M.D.
Taimur Zeb, M.D.
PL-2
Ricardo Calvo, M.D.
Lee N. Muecke, M.D.
Eduardo A. Otero, M.D.

Cynthia J. Hamilton, MD.
Terri A. Russell, M.D.

Eric N. Levy, M.D.
Donald K. Murphy, M.D.
Joanna K. Ramseyer-Weinberg, M.D.

PL-3
David L. Grundy, M.D.
Jayashree Mani, M.D.
Robert w. Weiting, III, M.D.

Eufrosina A.Y. Lua, M.D.
Monica Suchoff, M.D.

General Surgery
PL-3
Robert Alleyn, M.D.
John Sanders, M.D.

Michael Ratliff, M.D.
David Stalker, M.D.

PL-4
Elizabeth T. Bonefas, M.D.
Gary Kubalak, M.D.

Daniel Casso, M.D.
Dennis Meurer, M.D.

PL-5
Michael Coselli, M.D.

Jean-Pierre Forage, M.D.

HOUSE STAFF 1988-1989

Transitional Interns
Dale S. Glass, M.D.
Paul M. Lee, M.D.
Brett R. Ravkind, M.D.

David K. Harris, M.D.
Paul Metzger, III, M.D.
Machael S. Smith, M.D.

Family Practice
PL-1
David C. Carter, M.D.
Manuel J. Martin, M.D.
Doris. M. Robitaille, M.D.

Patricia S. Hanley, M.D,
Wendy M. Merola, M.D.
Bridget Robledo, M.D.

PL-2
James D. Behra, M.D.
Baldemar Covarrubias, M.D.
Horace G. Hinson, M.D.
Paul D. Keinarth, M.D.

Carol M. Byler, M.D.
Lisa B. Glenn, M.D.
David G. Joseph, M.D.

PL-3
Sylvia A. Adams, M.D.
Rebecca A. de la Torre, M.D.

Jeanne W. Cook, M.D.
Philip P. Huang, M.D.

Chief Res. 7/1/88-6/1/89
Jacqueline M. Kerr, M.D(). Walter R. Leverich, M.D.
Wail Malaty, M.D.

Internal Medicine
PL-1
Perer Cowley, M.D. Scott D. Meyer, M.D.
Leandro G. Pena, M.D. John B. Silman, M.D.
Edwin Woo, M.D.
PL-2
Rebecca Ellison, M.D. Carol Friedman, D.O.
Matthew E. Masters, M.D. Alina M. Ramos, M.D.
Terri T. Steele, M.D.
PL-3
Barbara A. Fedor, M.D. Maria R. Gallego, M.D.
Robert G. Huth, M.D.
Chief Res. 1/1/89-6/30/89 Mark A. Prange, M.D.
Darrell E. Wilburn, M.D. Harry S. Maxwell, M.D.
Chief Res. 7/1/-12/30/88

Pediatrics
PL-1
Elsa G. Brieno, M.D. Armando G. Correa, M.D.
Lamin f. Elerian, M.D. Dwayne E. Johnson, M.D.
Dhiraj a. Patel, M.D. Jesus E. Pina Garza, M.D.
PL-2
Alena Ashenberg, M.D. Cynthia J. Hamilton, M.D.
Truett A. Hull, M.D. Terri Anne RussellM.D.
Taimur Zeb, M.D.
PL-3
Eric M. Levy, M.D. Donald K. Murphy, M.D.
David C. Needham, M.D. Eduardo A. Otero, M.D.
Chief Res. 7/1/88-6/30/89
Joanna K. Ramseyer-
Weinberg, M.D. Robert W. Wieting, III, M.D.

Chief Res. 11/1/88-6/30/89

Surgery
PL-3
Dan Galvan, M.D.
Michael Sheridan, M.D.
PL-4
Robert Alleyn, M.D.
John Sanders, M.D.
PL-5
Elizabeth Bonefas, M.D.
Dennis Neurer, M.D.

Paul James, M.D.
Steven Thomas, M.D.

Michael Ratliff, M. D.
David Stalker, M.D.

Gary Kubalak, M.D.

HOUSE STAFF 1989-1990

Transitional Interns
Eugene N. Clayton, M.D.
Dione M. Garria, M.D.
David D. Moffat, M.D.

Eric J. Coligado, M.D.
Francisco Jaime, M.D.
Phillip A. Rinaldi, M.D.

Family Practice
PL-1
Horacio P. Guerra, M.D.
Michael E. Killian, M.D.
Nicholas A. Schroeder, M.D.
PL-2
David C. Carter, M.D.
Manuel J. Martin, M.D.
Doris M. Robitaille, M.D.
PL-3
James D. Behra, M.D.
Baldemar Covarrubias, M.D.
Horace G. Hinson, M.D.
Paul Keinarth, M.D.

Michael L. Gutierrez, M.D.
Gregg H. Lucksinger, M.D.
Yi Yang, M.D.

Patricia S. Hanley, M.D.
Wendy Merola, M.D.
Briget Robledo, M.D.

Carol M. Byler, M.D.
Lisa B. Glenn, M.D.
David G. Joseph, M.D.
Rebecca A. de la Torre, M.D.

Internal Medicine
PL-1
Stacei L. Bush-Veith, M.D.
James E. Lambeth, M.D.
Edwin Woo, D. O.
PL-2
James T. Gilley, M.D.
Leandro G. Pena, M.D.
John B. Silman, M.D.
PL-3
Rebecca Ellison, M.D.
Matthew E. Masters, M.D.
Terri t. Steele, M.D
Chief Res. 1/1/90-6/30/90
Chief Res. 7/1/-12/31/89

Paul J. Jennings, M.D
Helen J. Maidment, M.D.

Scott D. Meyer, M.D.
Brett R. Ravkind, M.D.

Carol Friedman, M.D.
Alina M Ramos, M.D.

Maria R. Gallego, M.D.

Pediatrics
PL-1
Sangeeta Agrawala, M.D.
Sriya W.C. Gunawardena, M.D.
Elana I Meza, M.D.
PL-2
Elsa B. Brieno, M.D.
Lamia F. Elerian, M.D.
Jesus E. Pina. M.D.
PL-3
Alena Ashenberg, M.D.
Terri Anne Russell, M.D.
PL-4 Instructor
Ricardo Calvo, M.D.

Diana R. Grave, M.D.
Javier R. Kane. M.D.
Luis Rodriguez, M.D.

Armando G. Correa, M.D.
Dwayne E. Johnson, M.D.

Truett a. Hull, M.D. Chief Res.
Taimur Zeb, M.D.

Surgery
PL-3
Donald Colins, M.D
Paula Oliver, M.D.

Can Galvan, M.D.
James Redfield, M.D.

PL-4
Paul James, M.D.   Michael Sheridan, M.D.
Bruce Smith, M.D.   Steven Thomas M.D.
PL-5
Robert Alleyn, M.D.   Michael Ratliff, M.D.
David Stalker, M.D.

HOUSE STAFF 1990-1991

Transitional Interns
Michael E. J. Archuleta, M.D.   Edward J. Burke, M.D.
David L. Craig, M.D.   Kianoush Kian, M.D.
Christopher Lam, M.D.   Michael T. Otte, M.D.

Family Practice
PL-1
Mary E. Bartz, M.D.   Cynthis C. Brinson, M.D.
James S. Hahn, M.D.   Wei-Ann Lin, M.D.
Kerry D. Rhodes, M.D.   Yi (Toney) Yang, M.D.
PL-2
Horacio P. Guerra, M.D.   Michael L. Gutierrez, M.D.
Gail S. Hovorka, M.D.   Michael E. Killian, M.D.
Gregg H. Lucksinger M.D.   Harvey Renger, Jr., M.D.
PL-3
David C. Carter, M.D.   Patricia S. Hanley, M.D.
Manuel J. Martin, M.D.   Wendy M. Merola, M.D. Chief
Doris M. Robitaille, M.D.   Bridget Robledo, M.D.

Internal Medicine
PL-1
Raymond B. Acebo, M.D.   Marilyn J. Friday, M.D.
Masoud Khorsand-Sahbaie, M.D.
Anelia T. Petkova, M.D.   Elaine A. Staten, D.O.
PL-2
Stacie L. Bush-Veith, M.D.   James E Lambeth, M.D.

Helen J. Maidment, M.D.
Edwin Woo, M.D.
PL-3
James T. Gilley, M.D.
Leandro G. Pena, M.D.
John B. Silman, M.D.
Chief resident

Connie L. Pham, M.D.

Scott D. Meyer, M.D.
Brett R. Ravkind, M.D.
Carol Griedman, D.O.
Chief resident

Pediatrics
PL-1
Nandini Kanagal, M.D.
Luis Rodriguez, M.D.
Swati D. Vora, M.D.
PL-2
Sangeeta Agrawala, MD.
Sriya W.C. Gunawardena, M.D.
Elena T. Meza, M.D.
PL-3
Elsa G. Briena, M.D.
Lamia F. Elerian, M.D.
Dwayne E. Johnson, M.D.

Maie D. Killian, M.D.
Vyjayanthi Srinivasan, M.D.

Diana R. Grave, M.D.
Javier R. Kane, M.D.

Armando G Correa, M.D.
Co-Cheif Resident
Jesus E. Pina, M.D. Co-Chief

Surgery
PL-2
Mark Hernandez, M.D
Carlton Perry, M.D.
PL-3
Kent Johnson, M.D.
John Williams, M.D.
PL-4
Donald Collins, M.D.
Paula Oliver, M.D.
PL-5
Paul James, MD.
Steven Thomas, M.D.

Jeffrey Meynig, M.D.
Jamie Terry, M.D.

Ben Mack, M.D.
Jeffrey Young, M.D.

Dan Galvan, M.D.
James Redfield, M.D.

Michael Sheridan, M.D.

HOUSE STAFF 1991-1992

Transitional Interns
Bonnie J Boenig, M.D.
Wade B. Etheredge, M.D.
Michael E. Pogodsky, M.D.
Anthony M. Deep, M.D.
Kathryn r. Hamilton, M.D.
William L. Preston, M.D.

Family Practice
James S. Gaertner, M. D.
Eun K. Kwun, M.D.
Laura K. Maurer, M.D.
John M. Haest, M.D.
Jill A. Litzinger, M.D.
Carmen P Wong, M.D.

Mary E. Bartz, M.D.
James S. Hahn, M.D.
Kerry D. Rhodes, M.D.
Cynthis C. Brinson, M.D.
Wei-Ann Lin, M.D.
Yi (Tony) Yang, M.D.

Noracio P. Guerra, M.D.
Gail S. Hovorka, M.D.
Gregg H. Lucksinger, M.D.
Chief Resident
Michael L. Gutierrez, M.D.
Michael E. Killian, M.D.
Harvey Renger, Jr. M.D.

Internal Medicine
John H. Lerma, M.D.
Irfan K. Sandozi, M.D.
Sarah I. Smiley, D. O.
Henry J. Lopez-Roman, M.D.
Donovan H. Sigerfoos, D.O.

Raymond B. Acebo, M.D.
Masoud Khorsand-Sahbaie, M.D.
Anelia T. Petkova, M.D.
Stacei L. Bush-Veith, M.D.
Helen J Maidment M.D.
Chief resident
Leandro g. Pena, M.D.
Chief Resident
Marilyn J. Friday, M.D.

Elaine A. Staten, D.O.
James E. Lambeth, M.D.
Connie L. Pham, M.D.
Edwin Woo, D.O.

Pediatrics

Asma A. Ahmad, M.D.
Houman Kiani, M.D.
Jose r. Reyes, M.D.

Binaca Gaglani, M.D.
Maria Melita Palasi, M.D.

Susan M. Goss, M.D.
Naie D. Killian, M.D.
Swati d. Vora, M.D.

Nandini Kanagal, M.D.
Luis Rodriguez, M.D.
Jeanne L. Wiegand, M.D.

Sangeeta Agrawala, M.D.
Sriya W.C. Gunawardena, M.D.
Elena I. Meza

Diana r. Grave, M.D.
Javier R. Kane, M.D.

Surgery

Michelle Bowman, M.D.
Joey Haber, M.D.

Alanna Craig, M.D.
Willie Melvin, M.D.

Mark Hernandez, M.D.
Carlton Perry, M.D.

Jeffrey Meynig, M.D.
Jamie Terry, M.D.

Kent Johnson, M.D.
John Williams, M.D.

Ben Mack, M.D.
Jeffrey Young, M.D.

Dan Galvan M.D.
James Redfield, M.D.

Paula Oliver, M.D.

HOUSE STAFF 1992-1993

Transitional Interns
Beto Alanis, M.D.
Ron Byrd, Jr, M.D.
Cary Gossett, M.D.

Harlan Bieley, M.D.
Chris Garrison, M.D.
Jim Michaels, M.D.

Family Practice
Roger Batlle, M.D.

Andre Chen, M.D.

Martha Coleman, M.D.
Joe McCreight, M.D.

Leigh Frednolm, M.D.
Claudia Molina Batlle, M.D.

Scott Gaertner, M.D.
Jeanine Kwun, M.D.
Carmen Wong, M.D.

John Haest, M.D.
Laura Maurer, M.D.

Mary Bartz, M.D.
Wei-Ann Lin, M.D.
Kerry Rhodes, M.D.
Cynthia Brinson, M.D.
Chief Resident

James Hahn, M.D.
Ann Messerm M.D.
Tony Yang, M.D.

Family Practice/ OB/Gyn. Fellows
Elizabeth Kinney, M.D.
Michelle Hagenbuch, M.D.

Internal Medicine
Suzan Arizpe, M.D.
Arifa Rahman, M.D.
Ziga Tretjak, M.D.

Aldo Parodi, M.D.
Vijoy Rao, M.D.
Tin Tin Wai, M.d.

Beth Bower, M.D.
John Lerma, M.D
Donovan Sigerfoos, M.D.

Shahzad Hasan M.D.
Henry Lopez-Roman, M.D
Sarah Smiley, M.D.

Raymond Acebo, M.D.
Masound Khorsand, M.D.
Anelin Petkova, M.D.
Chief Resident
Stacie Bush-Veith, M.D.
Chief Resident

Janice Friday, M.D.
Joe Mills, M.D.
Elaine Staten, M.D.

Pediatracs
Javier Gonzalez, M.D.

Daniel Manjarrez, MD.

Rafael Mimbela, M.D.
Jyortibala Ruparei, M.D.
Patricia Tenner, M.D.

Aquilla Moosani, M.D.
Asma Siddiqui, M.D

Asma Anmad, M.D.
Binaca Gaglani, M.D.

Anupama Bhardwaj, M.D.

Lauren Buxbaum, M.D.
Ayman Habiba, M.D.
Luis Rodriguez, M.D.
Jeanne Wiegand, M.D.
Chief Resident

Diana Grave, M.D.
Nandini Kanagal, M.D.
Swati Vora, M.D.
Susan Goss, M.D.

Surgery
Willie Melvin, M.D.
Jamie Terry, M.D.
Chief Resident

Jeff Meynig, M.D.
Kent Johnson, M.D.

HOUSE STAFF 1993-1994

Transitional Interns
Mark Crawford, M.D.
George Lyons, M.D.
Neuhoff, Robertson, M.D.
John Thompson, M.D.

Brian Kim, M.D.
Amy Rand, M.D.
Steve Robertson, M.D.

Family Practice
Marie Christensen, M.D.
Jennifer Speaker, M.D.
Kevin Stephens, M.D.

Michele LaRoe, M.D.
Dana Sprute, M.D.
Erika Zimmerman, M.D.

Roger Batlle, M.D.
Andre Chen, M.D.
Leigh Fredholm, M.D.

Ron Byrd, M.D.
Martha Coleman, M.D.
Joe McCreight, M.D.

Scott Gaertner, M.D.
Jeanine Kwun, M.D.
Laura Maurer, M.D.
Ann Messer, M.D.
Chief Resident

John Haest, M.D.
Jill Litzinger, M.D.
Carmen Wong, M.D.

Practice Ob-Gyn. Fellows
Edwin Herrera

Beta Harmon

Internal Medicine
Sofia Ayub, M.D.
Lawrence Chang, M.D.
Milton Shepperd, D.O.

Mike Brancheau, M.D.
Jorge Leiva, M.D.
Dash Wallooppillai, M.D.

Aldo Parodi, M.D.
Ziga Tretjak, M.D.

Vijoy Rao, M.D.
Tin Tin Wai, M.D.

Shahzad Hasan, M.D.
John Lerma, M.D.
Sara Smiley, D.O.
Donovan Sigerfoos, D.O.
Chief Resident

Larry Kotov, M.D.
Henry Lopez_Roman, M.D.
Wei-ming Tuan, M.D.

Pediatrics
Mariano Amador, M.D.
Helga Liptakova, M.D.
Luis Munoz, M.D.
Le-Wai Thant, M.D.

Marisol Fernandez, M.D.
Mitali Mitra, M.D.
Jyoti Ruparel, M.D.

Harminder Dhaliwal, M.D.
Javier Gonzalez, M.D.
Rafael Mimbela, M.D.
Ashraf Razak, M.D.

Cheryl Evans, M.D.
Daniel Manjarrez, M.D.
Aquilla Moosani, M.D.
Asma Siddiqui, M.D.

Asma Ahmad, M.D.

Joann Schulte, D.O.

Biaca Gaglani, M.D.
Chief Resident

Pediatric Emergency Medicine Fellow
Joanne G. Adams, M.D.

HOUSE STAFF 1994-1995

Transitional Interns
Bobby Hilliard, M.D.
Desmond Kidd, M.D.
James Lilly, M.D.

Andrea Jarma, M.D.
David Kim, M.D.
Wavne, Martin, M.D.

Family Practice
Juanita Bishop, M.D.
Sharon Hausman-Cohen, M.D.
Mindy Miller, M.D.
Denise Taylor, M.D.

Stephen Blair, M.D.
Mary Martinez, M.D.
Erica Moeller-Ruiz, M.D.

Marie Christensen, M.D.
Michele LaRoe, M.D.
Claudia Molina Batlle, M.D.
Dana Sprute, M.D.
Erika Zimmerman, M.D.

Steven Crow, M.D.
Roger Batlle, M.D.
Jennifer Speaker, M.D.
Kevin Stephens, M.D.

Ron Byrd, M.D.
Martha Coleman, M.D.
Joe McCreight, M.D.

Andre Chen, M.D.
John Haest, M.D.
Leigh Frednolm, M.D. Chief Res.

Family Practice/ Ob-Gyn Fellows
John Day, M.D.

Edwin Herrera, M.D.

Internal Medicine
Nuzhat Ahmed, M.D.
Franklin Chen, M.D.

Rajesh Bhandare, M.D.
Krzysztof Lyson, M.D.

Aruna Potti, M.D.
Carlos Rubin de Celis, M.D.

Deepa Ramaswamy, M.D.

Sofia Ayub, M.D.
Lawrence Chang, M.D.
Homero Salinas Perez, M.D.
Aruna Venkatesh, M.D.

Mike Brancheau, M.D.
Ricardo Garza, M.D.
Milton Shepperd, D.O.
Dash Wallooppillai, M.D.

Aldo Parodi, M.D.
Ziga Tretjak, M.D.
Wei-ming Tuan, M.D.
Chief resident

Vijoy Rao, M.D.
TinTin Wai, M.D.

Pediatrics
Omar Abuzaitoun, M.D.
Monica Farias, M.D.
Luz Elva Tristan, M.D.

Patricia Crowe, M.D.
Miguel Petrozzi, M.D.
Michael Walter, M.D.

Mariano Amador, M.D.
Marisol Fernandez, M.D.
Metali Mitra, M.D.
Jyoti Ruparel, M.D.

Harminder Dhaliwai, M.D.
Helga Liptakova, M.D.
Luis Munoz, M.D.
Le-Wai Thant, M.D.

Cheryl Evans, M.D.
Aquilla Moosani, M.D.
Asma Siddiqui, M. D.
Chief resident

Javier Gonzalez, M.D.
Anu Rao, M.D.
Daniel Manjarrez, M.D.

Pediatric Emergency Medicine Fellow
Joanne Gordon Adams, D.O.

HOUSE STAFF 1995-1996

Transitional Interns
Jeannie Hsu, M.D.

Kim Mulligan, M.D.

Brett Smith, M.D.
Kim Tran, M.D.

Chris Swanson, M.D.
David Wood, M.D.

Family Practice
Jennifer Arnecilla, M.D.
Jeff Hischke, M.D.
Vicki Miller, M.D.
Rachel Stover, M.D.

James Barbee. M.D.
Alex Marquis, M.D.
Rex Poole, M.D.

Steven Blair, M.D.
Mindy Miller M.D.
Denise Taylor, M.D.
Claudia Molina-Batlle, M.D.

Sharon Hausman-Cohen, M.D.
Erica Moeller-Ruiz, M.D.
Jennifer Huertas, M.D.

Marie Christensen, M.D.
Michele LaRoe, M.D.
Kevin Stephens, M.D.
Dana Sprute, M.D.
Chief resident

Steven Crow, M.D.
Jennifer Speaker, M.D.
Erika Zimmerman, M.D.

Internal Medicine
Kusum Bhandari, M.D.
Steven Cole, M.D.
Camille Hemlock, M.D.
Kim Rowland, M.D.
John Davidson, M.D.

Yurong Cai, M.D.
Maricarmen Fuentes, M.D.
Edwin McClelland, M.D.
Stanley Yang, M.D.
Roger Batlle, M.D.

Nuzhat Ahmed, M.D.
Franklin Chen, M.D.
Aruna Potti, M.D.
Camille Hemlock, M.D.

Rajesh Bhandari, M.D.
Krzysztof Lyson, M.D.
Carlos Rubin de Celis, M.D.
Kim Rowlands, M.D.

Sophia Ayub, M.D.
Lawrence Chang, M.D.
Homero Salinas-Perez, M.D.

Mike Brancheau, M.D.
Ricardo Garza, M.D.
Milton Shepperd, M.D.

Aruna Venkatesh, M.D.
Chief resident

Dash Wallooppillai, M.D.
Chief resident

Pediatrics

Pamela Atienza, M.D.
Sheila Boes, M.D.
Lucy Lot, M.D.
Vandana Mahajan, M.D.

Corinne Barber, M.D.
Mohammad Jarrar, M.D.
Helen Ma, M.D.

Omar Abuzaitoun, M.D.
Monica Farias, M.D.
Luz Elva Tristan, M.D.

Patricia Crowe, M.D.
Miguel Petrozzi, M.D.
Michael Walter, M.D.

Mariano Amador, M.D
Marisol Fernandez, M.D.
Mitali Mitra, M.D.
Jyoti Ruparel, M.D.
Javier Gonzalez, M.D.
Chief resident

Harminder Dhaliwal, M.D.
Helga Liptakova, M.D.
Luis Munoz, M.D.
Le-Wai Thant, M.D.

HOUSE STAFF 1996-1997

Transitional Interns

Tony Aldave, M.D.
Teresa Loftin, M.D.
Trent Turner, M.D.

Eric Hughes, MD.
Rick Roeske, M.D.
Kelly Van Epps. M.D.

Family Practice

Joshua DiCarlo, M.D.
Ralph Sharman, M.D.
Ryan Stallings, M.D.

Olufunke Ezekoye, M.D.
Stephen Shopbell, M.D
Tina Ward, M.D.

Jennifer Arnecillia, M.D.
Alex Marquis, M.D.
Rex Poole, M.D.

Jeffrey Hischke, M.D.
Vicki Miller, M.D.
Rachel Stover, M.D.

Kim Tran, M.D.

Stephen Blair, M.D.
Juanita Huertas, M.D.
Mary Martinez, M.D.
Erica Moeller-Ruiz, M.D.
Denise Taylor, M.D.
Pres, house staff assoc.

Sharon Hausman-Cohen, M.D.
Juanita Huertas, M.D. Chief res.
Mindy Miller, M.D.
Claudia Molina-Batlle, M.D.

Internal Medicine
Pratima K. Chhipa, M.D.
Nishani Gunasckera, M.D.
Teresa Lyson, M.D.
Lakshminaraya Ramakrishnan, M.D.
Raheela Sadiz, M.D.

Patrick Garcia, M.D.
Tareq Jamil, M.D.
Mujaddid Masood, M.D.

Kusum Bhandari, M.D.
John Davidson, M.D.
Maricarmen Fuentes, M.D.

Steve Cole, M.D.
Gina De Santo, M.D.
Stanley Yang, M.D.

Nuzhat Ahmed, M.D.
Mike Grancheau, M.D.
Camille Hemlock, M.D.
Aruna Potti, M.D.
Carlos Rubin de Celis, M.D.

Roger Batlle, M.D.
Franklin Chen, M.D.
Krzysztof Lyson, M.D.
Kim Rolands, M.D.

Rajesh Bhandari, M.D.
Chief resident

Pediatrics
Omar Al-Masri, M.D.
Mohamad Miqdady, M.D.
Toral Shah, M.D.
Suma Manjunath, M.D.

Fulgencio Braganza del Castillo,
Noel Nye, M.D.
Diana Stone, M.D.

Pamela Atienza, M.D.
Sheila Boes, M.D.
Lucy Lot, M.D.
Vandana Mahajan, M.D.

Corinne (Barber) West, D.O.
Mohammad Jarrar, M.D.
Helen Ma, D.O.

Omar Abuzaitoun, M.D.
Monica Farias, M.D.
Miguel Petrozzi M.D.

Patricia Crowe, M.D.
Michael Fischer, M.D.
Luz Elva Tristan, M.D.

Michael Walter, M.D.
Chief resident

Family Practice Ob/Gyn fellows
David R. Cesko, M.D.
Andrew Leuders, M.D.

Clark Craig, M.D.

HOUSE STAFF 1997-1998

Transitional Interns
John Campbell, M.D.
Vala Djafari, M.D.
Yvonne Queralt, M.D.

Mary Ana Cunningham, M.D.
David Hodge, M.D.
Chad Reder, M.D.

Family Practice
Melinda Astran, M.D.
Lance Carroll, M.D.
Jennifer Schroeder, M.D.
Tom Zavaleta, M.D.

Don Brode, M.D.
Yana Findelshteyn, M.D.
Alicia Wong, M.D.

J. W. Dailey, M.D.
Olfunke Ezekoye, M.D.
Stephen Shopbell, M.D.
Tina Ward. M.D.

Joshua DiCarlo, M.D.
Ralph sharman, M.D.
Ryan Stallings, M.D.

Jennifer Arnecillia, M.D.

Jeffrey Hischke, M.D.

Vicki Miller, M.D.
Rachel Stover, M.D.

Rex Poole, M.D.
Kim Tran, M.D.

Alex Marquis, M.D.
Chief resident

Internal Medicine

Jadranko Corak, M.D.
Octavia Graur, M.D.
Nioti Karim, M.D.
Mujahid Masood M.D.

Virginia Corpus, M.D.
Menaka Jayasundera, M.D.
James Kerbacher, M.D.
Robert Ramirez, M.D.

Mousumi Chandra-Kim, M.D.
Patrick Garcia, M.D.
Muaddid Masood, M.D.
Lakshmi Ramakrishnan, M.D.

Pratima K. Chhipa, M.D.
Tareeq Jamil, M.D.
Asma Nuri, M.D.
Raheela Sadiq, M.D.

Roger Batlle, M.D.
Steve Cole, D.O.
Gina DeSanto, M.D.
Jayasree Kailasam, M.D.

Kusum Bhandari, M.D.
John Davidson, M.D.
Maricarmen Fuentes, M.D.
Sanely Yang, M.D.

Carlos Rubindi Celis, M.D.
Chief resident

Pediatrics

Robert Gillespie, M.D.
Carmen Johnson, M.D.
Leonel Rodriguez, M.D.
Lakshmy Vaidyanathan, M.D.

Naveen Husain, M.D.
Nikki Primus, M.D.
Vicky Taylor, M.D.
Livania Zavala, M.D.

Omar Al-Masri, M.D.
Sangeeta Krishna, M.D.
Mohanad Miqdady, M.D.
Toral Shah, M.D.

Fulgencio del Castillo, M.D.
Suma Manjunath, M.D.
Noel Nye, D.O.

Pamela Atienza, M.D.
Lucy Lot, M.D.
Corinne West, D.O.

Mohammad Jarrar, M.D.
Helen Ma, D.O.

Sheila Boes, M.D. Chief resident
Vandana Mahajan, M.D. Chief resident

Family practice OB/Gyn. Fellows

Jesus Saucedo, M.D.
Michelle Shimizu, M.D.
Harry Yeates, M.D.

HOUSE STAFF 1998-1999

Transitional Interns
John Gray, M.D.
Joseph Lauro, M.D.
Todd Shepler, M.D.

Patrick Hooper, M.D.
Maria Rojas, M.D.
Thanh Van, M.D.

Family Practice
Sara Aderholt, M.D.
Derrick Garcia, M.D.
Julie Howard, M.D.
Thuy Nguyen-Doan, M.D.

Daniel Garcia, M.D.
Jane Glawe, M.D.
Julie Howard, M.D.
Stephen Thomas, M.D.

Melinda Astran, M.D.
Lance Carroll, M.D.
Jennifer Schroeder, M.D.
Tom Zavaleta, M.D.

Don Grode, M.D.
Yana Finkelshteyn, M.D.
Alicia Wong, M.D.

J.W. Dailey, M.D.
Ralph Sharman, M.D.
Tina Ward, M.D.

Olyfunke Exekoye, M.D.
Ryan Stallings, M.D.

Internal Medicine

Jaime Belmares-Avalos, M.D.
Flora Edision, M.D.
Amin Mery, M.D.
Pablo Molina, M.D.

Ksenija Corak, M.D.
Arshad Ghauri, M.D.
Deepa Mittal, M.D.
Ruben Pipek, M.D.

Jadranko Corak, M.D.
Grag Gonzaba, M.D.
Nioti Karim, M.D.
Durba Mishra, M.D.

Virginia Corpus, M.D.
Menaka Jayasundera, M.D.
Mujahid Masood, M.D.
Robert Ramirez, M.D.

Sumi Chanda-Kim, M.D.
Tareq jamil, M.D.
Mujaddid Masood, M.D.
Lakshmi Ramakrishnan, M.D.

Patrick Garcia, M.D.
Pratima Kumar M.D.
Asma Nuri, M.D.
Raheela sadiq, M.D.

John Davidson, M.D. Chief resident.

Pediatrics

Jeffrey Alvis, M.D.
Juanita Bhatnagar, M.D.
Dominique Isenhower, M.D.
Nelson Spinetti, M.D.

Melecio Apostol, M.D.
Liz Harvey, M.D.
Paul Quesada, M.D.
Kelly Thorstad, M.D.

Robert Gillesie, M.D.
Carmen Johnson, M.D.
Nikki Primus, M.D.
Vicky Taylor, M.D.
Livania Zavala, M.D.

Naveen Husain, M.D.
Sangeeta Krishna, M.D.
Leonel Rodriguez, M.D.
Lakshmy Vaidyanathan, M.D.

Omar al-Masri, M.D.
Mohamad Miqdady, M.D.
Corinne West, D.O.

Fugencio Del Castillo, M.D.
Torl Shah, M.D.

Family Practice Ob/Gyn. Fellows
Suma Manjunath, M.D.　　　　Noel Nye, D.O.

HOUSE STAFF 1999-2000

Transitional Interns,
Darcey Bittner, M.D.　　　　Lance Carroll, M.D.
Carina Lawson, M.D.　　　　Gregory Connor, M.D.
Shawn Laney, M.D.　　　　Elizabeth Seaberg, M.D.

Family Practice
Earl J. Clement II, M.D.　　　　Todd Crump, M.D.
Danielle Eigner, M.D.　　　　Donald Simmons, M.D.
Mingsheng Tang, M.D.　　　　Brian Williams, M.D.
David Young, M.D.

Sarah Aderholt, M.D.　　　　Daniel Garcia, M.D.
Derrick Garcia, M.D.　　　　Jane Glawe, M.D.
Julie Howard, M.D.　　　　Thuy Nguyen-Doan, M.D.
Stephen Thomas, M.D.

Melinda Astran, M.D.　　　　Yana Finkelshteyn, M.D.
Jennifer Schroeder, M.D.　　　　Ryan Stallings, M.D.
Alicia Wong, M.D.　　　　Tom Zavaleta, M.D.
Don Brode, M.D.　　　　Lance Carroll, M.D.
Chief resident　　　　Chief resident

Internal Medicine
Daniela Drosu, M.D.　　　　Hien Duong, D.O.
Penelope Gonzalez, MD.　　　　Patrick Haskell, D.O.
Bharathi Kondur, M.D.　　　　Huifang Lu, M.D.
Behzad Mosharafian, M.D.　　　　Ann Shippy, M.D.
David Winkler, M.D.

Jamie Belmares-Avalos, M.D.　　　　Ksenija Corak, M.D.
Flora Edison M.D.　　　　Arshad Ghauri, M.D.

Amin Mery, M.D.
Pablo Molina, M.D.

Jadranko Corak, M.D.
Greg Gonzaba, M.D.
Nioti Karim, M.D.
Durba Mishra, M.D.
Raheela Sadiq, M.D.

Patrick Garcia, M.D.
Chief resident

Deepa Mittal, M.D.
Ruben Pipek, M.D.

Virginia Corpus, M.D
Menaka Jayasundera, M.D.
Mujahid Massood, M.D.
Robert Ramirez, M.D.

Pediatrics
David Askenazi, M.D.
Miguel Moreno, M.D.
Franscene Oulds, M.D.
Robert Vezzetti, M.D.

Shawn Hathaway, M.D.
Barbie Norman, M.D.
Kathleen Powderly, M.D.
Sara Woods, M.D.

Jeffrey Alvis, M.D.
Juanita Bhatnagar, M.D.
Dominique Isenhower, M.D.
Paul Quesada, M.D.
Kelly thorstad, M.D.

Melecio Apostol, M.D.
Liz Holliman, M.D.
Dayo Lanier, M.D.
Nelson Spinetti, M.D.
Tibisay Villalobos, M.D.

Robert Gillespie, M.D.
Nikki Primus, M.D.
Toral Shah, M.D.
Lakshmy Vaidyanathan, M.D.

Naveen Husain, M.D.
Leonel Rodriguez, M.D.
Vicky Taylor, M.D.

Carmen Johnson, M.D.
Chief resident

Livania Zavala, M.D.
Chief resident

Family Practice Ob//gyn. Fellows
Derrick Cameron, M.D.
Cassandra Garcia, M.D.
Lisa Clemons, M.D.

Nathan Eliason, M.D.
Deborah Glupczynski, M.D.
Kristi Norris, M.D.

Appendix B

Interns and residents that rotated through the Austin Bone and Joint Clinic.
The office in which the author practiced.

Family practice

Douglas Wohlfahrt, MD
Constance Hanna, MD
Walter R. Leverich, MD
Doris Robitaille, MD
Baldemar Covarrubias, MD
Paul Keinarth, MD
Cynthis Brinson, MD
James Hahn, MD
Mary Bartz, MD
Ann Messer, MD
James S. Gaertner, MD
Leigh Fredholm, MD
Roger Batlle, MD
Marie Christensen, MD
Sharon Housman-Cohen, MD
Steven Blair, MD
Olufunke Ezekoye, MD
Stephen Shoppbell, MD

Lynn Warthan, MD
David Wright, MD
David C. Carter, MD
Patricia Hanley, MD
Mike Killian, MD
Gregg Lucksinger, MD
Yi (Toney) Yang, MD
Wei-Ann Lin, MD
Kerry Rhodes, MD
Carmen Wong, MD
Laura Mauer, MD
Martha Coleman, MD
Erika Zimmerman, MD
Kevin Stephenson, MD
Erica Moeller-Ruiz, MD
Vickie Miller, MD
Rachael Stover, MD
Ryan Stallings, MD

Tina Ward, MD
Tom Zavaleta, MD
Kim Tran, MD
J. W. Dailey, MD
Todd Crump, MD
Donald Simmons, MD
David Young, MD
Brian Williams, MD
Do Keng, MD
Jason Nurnberg, MD
Bovert Sanchez, MD
Eric Arhelger, MD

Melinda Astran, MD
Yana Findelshteyn, MD
Jennifer Schroeder, MD
Derrick Garcia, MD
Jane Glawe, MD
Steve Thomas, MD
Gala Trickey, MD
Sekou Ford, MD
Koy In, MD
Margaret Brown, MD
Veronica Ruiz, MD

Internal medicine residents

Mike Brancheau, MD
Lawrence Chang, MD
Nuzhat Ahmed, MD
Carlos Rubindi Celis, MD
Christoff Lyson, MD
Roger Batlle, MD
Jasaree Kailasem, MD
Maricarmen Fuentes, MD
Tin TinWai, MD
Sumi Shandra-Kim, MD
Robert Ramirez, MD
Minaha Jayasurdia, MD
Deepra Mitlal, MD
Daniella Drosu, MD
Rosanie Valyasivi, MD
Daniel Shih, MD
Husna Musa, MD

Homero Salinas, Perez, MD
Milton Sheppard, MD
Aruna Potti, MD
Kim Roulands, MD
Camille Hemlock, MD
Gina DeSantos
Kusum Bhandari, MD
Lakshmi Ramakrishnan, MD
Mujaddid Masood, MD
Moite Karim, MD
Durba Mishra, MD
Pablo Molina, MD
Mary Amin, MD
Ann Shippy, MD
Christian Cipleu, MD
Kan Liu, MD
Matt Hill, MD

ARTICLES OF INCORPORATION

OF

THE CENTRAL TEXAS MEDICAL FOUNDATION

We, the undersigned natural persons of the age of twenty-one (21) years or more, at least two of whom are citizens of the State of Texas, acting as incorporators of an incorporation under the Texas Non-Profit Corporation Act, do hereby adopt the following Articles of Incorporation for such corporation:

ARTICLE ONE

The name of the corporation is THE CENTRAL TEXAS MEDICAL FOUNDATION.

ARTICLE TWO

The corporation is a non-profit corporation.

ARTICLE THREE

The period of its duration is perpetual.

ARTICLE FOUR

The purposes for which the corporation is organized and its powers are:

(a) To promote, develop, define and encourage medical education and the distribution of medical health services and care by its members to the people of Travis County and the Central Texas area; to protect the public health; to provide for the delivery of medical and health care; to work and study with all legally constituted agencies and plans; to upgrade and sustain good medical care. To work with legally constituted governmental agencies and the general public, and with its legal representatives, employers and employees associations and other groups and individuals as to the availability of adequate medical care; to work in conjunction with the Travis County Medical Society and other societies and associations dedicated to the betterment of health care; to promote these purposes and the purposes to those organizations namely: the development the protection of public health; to accept gifts, trusts, and donations; and to receive property by devise and bequests.

(b) To supervise, manage and administer for its members, any medical, health, educational and service plans which involve, but are not limited to health and medical services under group insurance policies or contracts, medical or hospital service agreements, membership or subscription contracts and other similar group arrangements.

(c) To foster, encourage and coordinate the establishment of uniform standards of medical care and health services amongst other similar foundations.

(d) To establish for and on behalf of its members and the general public a standard uniform procedure and schedule by which any individual receiving medical or health service and care will have the opportunity of a fair hearing or any dispute or grievance in relation thereto.

(e) To keep, collect, maintain, record and preserve records and statistical information of all its members as the same may relate to all programs for medical care and the purposes of this foundation.

(f) To negotiate, enter into, make, perform, and carry out contracts of every kind for any lawful purpose with any person, firm, association, corporation, municipality, government, state territory, country or other municipal or government subdivision.

(g) To purchase, acquire, own, hold, lease either as lessee or as lessor, sell, exchange, mortgage, deed in trust, develop, construct, maintain, equip, operate, and generally deal in real property and other buildings and any and all property of any and every kind or description, whether real, personal, or mixed. Subject to Part Four, Texas Miscellaneous Laws Act.

(h) From time to time to apply for, purchase, acquire, transfer, or otherwise exercise, carry out, and enjoy any benefit, right, privilege, prerogative, or power conferred by, acquired under, or granted by any statute, ordinance, order, license, power, authority, franchise, commission, right, or privilege which any government or authority or governmental agency or corporation or other public body may be empowered to enact, make or grant.

(i) To perform and carry on any activity whatsoever which this foundation may deem proper or convenient in connection with any of the foregoing purposes, or which may be calculated directly or indirectly to promote the interests of this foundation or to enhance or further the accomplishment of any of its powers, purposes, and objects; to conduct its business in this state, and in other states, and in the District of Columbia, the territories of the United States, and in foreign countries; and to hold, purchase, mortgage, and convey real and personal property either in or out of the State of Texas, and to have and to exercise all the powers conferred by the laws of the State of Texas upon corporations formed under the laws pursuant to and under which this corporation is formed, as such laws are now in effect or may at any time hereafter be amended.

(j) To carry out all or any part of the foregoing objects and purposes as principal, agent, or otherwise, either alone or in conjunction with any person, firm, association, or other corporations and in any part of the world; and for the purpose of attaining or furthering any of its objects or purposes, to make and perform such contracts of any kind and description, to do such acts and things, and to exercise any and all such powers, as a natural person could lawfully make, perform, do, or exercise, provided that the same shall not be inconsistent with the laws of the State of Texas.

The foregoing statements of purposes shall be construed as a statement of both purposes and powers, and the purpose and powers stated in each clause shall, except where otherwise expressed, be in no way limited or restricted by reference to or inference from the terms or provisions of any other clause, but shall be regarded as independent purposes.

ARTICLE FIVE

The street address of the initial registered offices of the corporation is 4300 North Lamar Boulevard, Austin, Texas 78756, and the name of the initial registered agent at such address is John N. Kemp.

ARTICLE SIX

The number of trustees shall not be less than nine (9) nor more than seventeen (17). The number of trustees constituting the initial Board of Trustees of the Corporation is twelve (12) and the names of the persons who are to serve as initial Trustees are:

Darrell B. Faubion, M. D. - 105 Medical Park Tower, Austin, Texas
Hardy E. Thompson, M. D. - 910 West 19th Street, Austin, Texas
Grover L. Bynum, M. D. - 601 Medical Park Tower, Austin, Texas
H. S. Arnold, M. D. - 1010 West 40th Street, Austin, Texas
Robert A. Dennison, M. D. - 102 Medical Park Tower, Austin, Texas
Robert F. Ellzey, M. D. - 113 Medical Park Tower, Austin, Texas
Sam N. Key, Jr., M. D. - 606 Medical Park Tower, Austin, Texas
Morris D. McCauley, M. D. - 706 West 19th Street, Austin, Texas
G. Clifford Thorne, M. D. - #12 Medical Arts Square, Austin, Texas
Albert F. Vickers, M. D. - 1301 Nueces, Austin, Texas
John R. Rainey, Jr., M. D. - #8 Medical Arts Square, Austin, Texas
James M. Graham, M. D. - 202 Medical Park Tower, Austin, Texas

ARTICLE SEVEN

The name and street address of each incorporator is:

Darrell B. Faubion, M. D. - 105 Medical Park Tower, Austin, Texas
Hardy E. Thompson, M. D. - 910 West 19th Street, Austin, Texas
Grover L. Bynum, M. D. - 601 Medical Park Tower, Austin, Texas

ARTICLE EIGHT

This Foundation shall conduct and carry on its business without profit to itself or to its members, or any class thereof. No member shall, by reason of membership herein, be or become entitled at any time to receive any assets, property, income, or earnings from the Foundation or to profit therefrom in any manner.

ARTICLE NINE

In case of the liquidation, dissolution, or winding up of the corporation, whether voluntary or involuntary, or by operation of law, the assets and properties of the corporation shall be distributed and disposed of by the Board of Trustees of the corporation in furtherance of exempt purposes to a non-profit charitable, educational, or scientific organization which is itself exempt, or to the State of Texas or a local political subdivision of the State of Texas.

IN WITNESS WHEREOF, we have hereunto set our hands this the ____ day of _____, A. D. 1972.

_____
Darrell B. Faubion, M. D.

_____
Hardy E. Thompson, M. D.

_____
Grover L. Bynum, M. D.

THE STATE OF TEXAS |
COUNTY OF TRAVIS |

    I, *Harriett K. Clark*, a Notary Public, do hereby certify that on the *2nd* day of *May*, 1972, personally appeared Darrell B. Faubion, M. D., who being by me first duly sworn, declared that he is the person who signed the foregoing document as Incorporator, and that the statements therein contained are true.

    IN WITNESS WHEREOF, I have hereunto set my hand and seal the day and year above written.

                             Harriett K. Clark
                            Notary Public in and for Travis County, Texas

THE STATE OF TEXAS |
COUNTY OF TRAVIS |

    I, *Harriett K. Clark*, a Notary Public, do hereby certify that on the *2nd* day of *May*, 1972, personally appeared Hardy E. Thompson, M. D., who being by me first duly sworn, declared that he is the person who signed the foregoing document as Incorporator, and that the statements therein contained are true.

    IN WITNESS WHEREOF, I have hereunto set my hand and seal the day and year above written.

                             Harriett K. Clark
                            Notary Public in and for Travis County, Texas

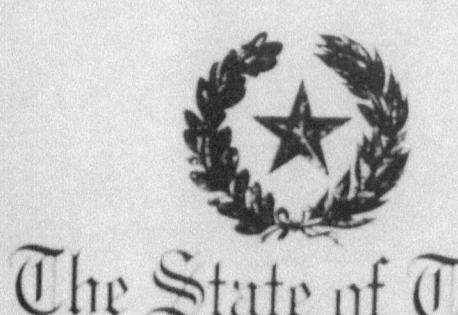

The State of Texas

SECRETARY OF STATE

The undersigned, as Secretary of State of the State of Texas, HEREBY CERTIFIES that the attached is a true and correct copy of the following described instruments on file in this Office:

THE CENTRAL TEXAS MEDICAL FOUNDATION

Articles of Incorporation

May 3, 1972

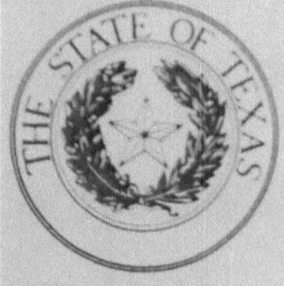

IN TESTIMONY WHEREOF, I have hereunto signed my name officially and caused to be impressed hereon the Seal of State at my office in the City of Austin, this 16th day of April A. D. 1990

Secretary of State

REVISED MINUTES OF THE MEMBERSHIP MEETING
OF THE
CENTRAL TEXAS MEDICAL FOUNDATION
JANUARY 28, 1998

A specially called meeting of the membership of the Central Texas Medical Foundation was called to order by James D. Lindley, M.D., President at 6:30 p.m. in the Thompson Auditorium at the Texas Medical Association Headquarters Building, 401 West 15th Street, Austin, Texas 78701. Sixty-three members were present at the meeting and 58 proxies were submitted prior to the meeting and were certified as valid. The Secretary certified that quorum was present.

Proposed transfer of Central Texas Medical Foundation to CTMF, Inc. The purpose of the meeting was to consider and vote on the transfer of assets of the graduate medical education program of the Central Texas Medical Foundation to CTMF, Inc. Dr. Lindley presented details of the proposed transaction to the membership. Dr. James Lindsey represented CTMF, Inc. and discussed the transaction from the Purchaser's point of view.

Action: Motion was made and seconded to adopt the following Resolution:

RESOLVED, that the membership of the Central Texas Medical Foundation authorize the sale and transfer of the graduate medical education program and the assets of that program, and the name "Central Texas Medical Foundation", to CTMF, Inc. and that the President of the of the Central Texas Medical Foundation be authorized to execute such documents and approve the Purchase Agreement in order to consummate the sale and transfer, and further that the Foundation change its name to the "Travis County Medical Society Foundation".

The Resolution was approved by a vote of 118 to 3.

There being no further business, the meeting was adjourned.

Attested by:

[signature]

James R. Brown, M.D., Secretary

As Custodian of the Records of the Central Texas Medical Foundation, I hereby certify the above is true and correct a portion of the membership meeting of the Central Texas Medical Foundation, January 28, 1998.

[signature]

Marshall Cothran, Executive Director
Central Texas Medical Foundation
Dated: 8/13/98

www.ingramcontent.com/pod-product-compliance
Lightning Source LLC
Chambersburg PA
CBHW020745180526
45163CB00001B/357